# AN INTRODUCTION TO PERFORMANCE ANALYSIS OF SPORT

Performance analysis has become an essential tool for coaches, athletes, sports organisations and academic researchers. Collecting and interpreting performance data enables coaches to improve their training programmes, athletes to make better tactical decisions, sports organisations to manage teams more effectively, and researchers to develop a better understanding of sports performance. This book is an essential introduction to the fundamental principles of performance analysis of sport and how to develop and operate performance analysis systems.

Containing worked examples from real sporting events throughout, the book introduces the basics of quantitative and qualitative performance analysis, reviews the different types of data and information that performance analysis can generate, and explains how to test for reliability. It presents a step-by-step guide to developing both manual and computerised analysis systems, and writing up and presenting findings from performance analysis programmes. Representing the most up-to-date, concise and engaging introduction to sports performance analysis, this book is an ideal course text for all introductory performance analysis courses, as well as an invaluable primer for coaches and practitioners in sport.

**Peter O'Donoghue** is Reader and Discipline Director for Performance Analysis in the Cardiff School of Sport, Cardiff Metropolitan University, UK. He is a member of the International Society of Performance Analysis of Sport, editor of the *International Journal of Performance Analysis of Sport*, and editor of the book series *Routledge Studies in Sports Performance Analysis*. He has extensive experience of providing performance analysis support in elite sport, and his research interests include relative age distribution in sport, predictive modelling of sports performance, and strategy in elite racket sport competition.

# Routledge Studies in Sports Performance Analysis

Series Editor
Peter O'Donoghue
*Cardiff Metropolitan University*

*Routledge Studies in Sports Performance Analysis* is designed to support students, lecturers and practitioners in all areas of this important and rapidly developing discipline. Books in the series are written by leading international experts in sports performance analysis and cover topics including match analysis, analysis of individual sports and team sports, technique analysis, data analytics, performance analysis for high performance management, and various methodological areas. Drawing on the very latest research, and introducing key concepts and best practice, the series meets a need for accessible, up-to-date texts at all levels of study and work in performance analysis.

Available in this series:

**An Introduction to Performance Analysis of Sport**
*Peter O'Donoghue*

# AN INTRODUCTION TO PERFORMANCE ANALYSIS OF SPORT

PETER O'DONOGHUE

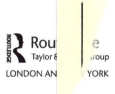

Routledge
Taylor & Francis Group

LONDON AND NEW YORK

First published 2015
by Routledge
2 Park Square, Milton Park, Abingdon, Oxon OX14 4RN

and by Routledge
711 Third Avenue, New York, NY 10017

*Routledge is an imprint of the Taylor & Francis Group, an informa business*

*British Library Cataloguing-in-Publication Data*
A catalogue record for this book is available from the British Library

*Library of Congress Cataloging-in-Publication Data*
O'Donoghue, Peter.
An introduction to performance analysis of sport / Peter O'Donoghue.
pages cm — (Routledge studies in sports performance analysis)
Includes bibliographical references and index.
1. Sports—Physiological aspects. 2. Sports sciences—Research.
3. Performance—Research. I. Title.
RC1235.O36 2015
613.7'1072—dc 3
2014013321

ISBN: 978-0-415-73985-6 (hbk)
ISBN: 978-0-415-73986-3 (pbk)
ISBN: 978-1-315-81634-0 (ebk)

Typeset in Melior and Univers
by FiSH Books Ltd, Enfield

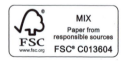

Printed and bound by CPI Group (UK) Ltd, Croydon, CR0 4YY

**To Zsófia**

# CONTENTS

# LIST OF FIGURES

ix

**list of figures**

# LIST OF TABLES

**list of tables**

# ACKNOWLEDGEMENTS

This book has been specifically developed for use by Level 5 (second year) degree students who are taking a sports performance analysis module. I would like to thank my colleagues at Cardiff Metropolitan University who deliver this module: Darrell Cobner, Adam Cullinane, Lucy Holmes, Ray Ponting and Huw Wiltshire. There are sports students who I have supervised over the last 18 years who have done projects that have inspired the examples used in this book. Specifically, Jonny Bloomfield, Emily Brown, Peter Clark, Lloyd Evans, Nicholas Harries, Philip Hunter, Dianne Liddle, Michael McCorry, Rhys Morgan, Ben Moss, Venkat Narayn, Scott Over and Gemma Robinson have done excellent work that has been thought provoking for the sports performance analysis discipline. I would also like to thank William Bailey, Josh Wells and Simon Whitmore from Routledge for their assistance during the planning and developing of this book.

Thank you all.

# CHAPTER 1

## WHAT IS SPORTS PERFORMANCE ANALYSIS?

### INTRODUCTION

This introductory chapter introduces sports performance analysis by asking the following questions: What? Why? Who? Where? When? and How? What is sports performance analysis? What are sports performance data and information? Why do we analyse sports performance? Who analyses sports performance? Where is sports performance analysis done? When is sports performance analysis done? How is sports performance analysis done? The answers to these questions are not independent. The reason why sports performance analysis is done and who requires the information can dictate what information is required. The information required can in turn influence when it is needed and thus when sports performances should be analysed. The time at which information is needed and economic constraints dictate the methods and locations of sports performance analysis tasks. These questions will be answered in turn but readers can expect some necessary overlap between the answers.

This chapter recognises that sports performance analysis is primarily an observational analysis task. The reason for doing it is to improve sports performance although there are also rehabilitation, academic, media and judging contexts of sports performance analysis. The roles of players, coaches and analysts with respect to data gathering and feedback within the coaching process are discussed. Sports performance analysis can be done at match venues, performance analysis laboratories and other locations. There are sports performance analysis activities that are done before, during and after competition, and the chapter distinguishes between live during-match analysis and post-match analysis. The final question is 'How?' This is answered by introducing the main manual and computerised methods that will be covered in detail later in the book.

Another way of phrasing the question 'What?' is by asking 'What should be analysed?' Specifically, what are the purposes of using sports performance analysis and what aspects of sports performance can be analysed. There are many different purposes of sports performance analysis including analysis of players, teams, coach behaviour and referees (O'Donoghue, 2010: 4–5). The purposes include work-rate analysis (Carling and Bloomfield, 2013), tactical analysis (Hibbs and O'Donoghue, 2013), effectiveness of chosen techniques (Palao and Morante, 2013) and analysis of technique (Lees, 2008; Campos, 2013). Academic investigations are done into factors influencing sports performance (Taylor *et al.*, 2008; Gomez *et al.*, 2013). There are also judging (Kirkbride, 2013a) and media (James, 2008; Kirkbride, 2013b) applications of sports performance analysis. This chapter includes a section on two main purposes of sports performance analysis that will be used throughout this book; work-rate analysis and match analysis. The match analysis purpose combines tactical analysis with analysing the effectiveness of skills. This is because tactical choices can be evaluated by how effectively they are applied.

## SPORTS PERFORMANCE ANALYSIS: WHAT? WHY? WHO? WHERE? WHEN? AND HOW?

### What is sports performance analysis?

This is the first of three subsections asking the question 'What?' in relation to sports performance analysis; what is sports performance analysis, what are the purposes of sports performance analysis and what variables should be analysed? In considering what sports performance analysis is, we are considering the nature of the sports performance analysis in practice as well as the academic discipline.

The main thing that distinguishes sports performance analysis from other disciplines of sports science is that actual performance is analysed. This is usually done through observation of the performance which could be live or post-competition if it has been video recorded. Sports performance analysis would typically not include either of the following:

2

- Self-report studies such as interviews, focus groups or questionnaires that explore general motives, intentions, attitudes and beliefs about sport.
- Laboratory experiments, field experiments or testing.

However, O'Donoghue (2010: 2) proposed that self-report and laboratory methods could be included within the scope of sports performance analysis under certain conditions. Any data coming from actual sports performance allows studies to fall within the broad scope of sports performance analysis. Such data are not limited to observational data. The data can include qualitative data, quantitative data, notation, video sequences, measurement, heart-rate responses, perceived exertion, blood lactate measures, EEG (electroencephalography) measures and EMG (electromyography) measures. Measurements of acceleration and location are possible during sports performance. Location can be sampled at 10Hz or greater by devices that can be worn by players during training and that are permitted during competition in some sports. There are thoughts and decision making processes that occur during actual sports performance that cannot be directly observed but which are relevant aspects of sports performance. Where an athlete observes a recording of their performance, reflecting on it and discusses the thoughts they had and decisions they made during the performance, interview data allow this aspect of performance to be studied (Poziat et al., 2010). This is a different use of self-report techniques to their traditional use in researching general attitudes and beliefs. It is an innovative use of interviews, focus groups, accounts or other self-report methods to investigate the experience of actual sports performance.

There is a case to be made for some controlled laboratory experiments falling within the scope of sports performance analysis. Analysis of technique has been done using biomechanics methods (Bartlett, 1999; Lees, 2008). Although many biomechanics investigations are done away from actual competition and training, biomechanics techniques have long been recognised as being within the scope of performance analysis (Hughes and Bartlett, 2004, 2008). Technique is an important aspect of sport, especially in cyclic sports activities such as running, swimming, cycling and walking (Marinho et al., 2013) as well as explosive sports such as field events in athletics (Campos, 2013). Lees (2008) classified skills as event skills, major skills and minor skills. Event skills constitute the entire event being performed such as the long jump. Major skills are dominant skills in the given sport, for example hurdling in sprint hurdles. Minor skills are important skills performed in the sport which are not dominant. There are games that contain critically important techniques such as the golf swing or the tennis serve. It is often not possible to collect detailed information about technique during actual competition. Setting up, calibrating and using a system such as Vicon™ (Vicon, Los Angeles, CA) on the first tee of the Ryder Cup or on Centre Court at Wimbledon is not going to happen. Therefore, important skills of sports are analysed in laboratory situations. While this is not actual competition and the limitations are recognised, relevant skills of the sport such as running stride, golf swing and tennis serve are being examined. Often there is a trade-off between ecological validity and experimental control. Ecological validity is where the study is representative of the real world context of interest. Observing actual sports performance has strong ecological validity. However, actual sports performance is not controlled by analysts and is influenced by many factors. Therefore, experimental control is not possible when studying actual competition. Laboratory studies of technique can be done under controlled conditions while also having a reasonable degree of ecological validity due to the importance and frequency with which the skills under investigation occur within competition.

**What are the application areas of sports performance analysis?**

The second 'What' is 'What are the application areas of sports performance analysis?' There are coaching, media, judging and academic purposes. Within a coaching context, sports performance analysis is used within a cycle of competing, reflecting, decision making and preparing for further competition (Franks, 1997; O'Donoghue and Mayes, 2013a). In practical situations within coaching environments, training is analysed as well as performance (Winkler, 1988; Mayes *et al.*, 2009). The term 'feed-forward' has been used instead of feedback where performance is analysed during training (Dowrick and Raeburn, 1977; Dowrick, 1991). Much of the research on feed-forward has focused on individual techniques. The purpose of analysing closed skills in detail within laboratory situations is to rehearse and improve these prior to competition. Feed-forward has also been applied in games sports with documented examples going back to 20 years. Consider the video of the England Football Squad's qualifying campaign for the 1994 World Cup ('Do I Not

4

Like That!'). One of the interesting sections in this video was the coverage of the home qualifying match against Poland. The video interleaved excerpts from a training session prior to this match with footage from the actual match which England won by three goals to nil. In one part, it shows the head coach, Graham Taylor, warning that Poland's defence was vulnerable when dealing with crosses and that crosses should be played in early to England's centre forward, Les Ferdinand. The squad were shown playing crosses in training with forwards running into the penalty area to head the ball towards goal. Then the video showed where this was successfully done in the match with Les Ferdinand heading a goal from a cross. Another part showed Paul Gascoigne, Stuart Pearce and Graham Taylor discussing a way of taking a free kick if Poland set up a defensive wall. This was rehearsed in training and the programme also showed this type of free kick being used by Stuart Pearce to score a goal in the match. These are examples of feed-forward, because they allow areas of performance to be analysed before the match and decisions to be made about how to play. These decisions may involve abandoning tactics that the team cannot perform successfully, or selecting players who can effectively implement the tactics that have been rehearsed.

In an academic context, sports performance analysis is used to research many areas of sports performance. There are investigations that use exclusively observational methods, while others use sports performance analysis as part of a multi-disciplinary investigation allowing use of complementary methods. Examples of studies that have used computerised notational analysis along with qualitative techniques include some studies of coach behaviour that have been done using the Arizona State University Observation Instrument (ASUOI) (Lacy and Darst, 1984, 1985, 1989). One study of netball coach behaviour used the ASUOI to compare coaches of different levels and then presented these results to an expert coach who was interviewed about the differences between coaches of different levels (Donnelly and O'Donoghue, 2008). Another example of sport performance analysis being used with other methods was a triangulation of computerised time-motion analysis of netball performance, psychological inventory and interviews (Hale, 2004). Hale compared competitive matches with training matches played by seven players using computerised time-motion analysis, having asked the players to complete the DM-CSAI2 questionnaire before the matches. After the matches, players were interviewed about the experiences of playing in training and competitive matches.

Lupo *et al.* (2012) used time-motion analysis and physiological measures to assess the demands of waterbasket. Larkin *et al.* (2011) investigated Australian Rules football using performance analysis to identify situations to include in a system used to test game understanding of players and umpires. The system was used within a prediction task which was developed into a test protocol used by players and umpires. Robinson *et al.* (2011) undertook a triangulation study to evaluate the risk associated with player movements in FA Premier League soccer. Time-motion analysis was triangulated with anthropometric measures and injury history data. The number of sharp path changes to the left, right and V-cut path changes were analysed over a series of six or more matches per player and compared between players who had missed matches or training days through injury and those who had not. It was found that taller, heavier players tended to perform fewer path changes than smaller, lighter players.

In this section of the chapter, we have not covered the refereeing and media applications of sports performance analysis, but these will be covered when considering 'Who' uses sports performance analysis.

## What do we analyse within sports performances?

As well as considering what performance analysis is and its broad application purposes, we also need to consider what aspects of performance should be analysed. This is a third 'What'. The purposes of performance analysis of sport (Hughes, 1998; O'Donoghue, 2010) are:

- Analysis of technique
- Analysis of effectiveness
- Tactical analysis
- Movement analysis
- Analysis of decision making

Analysis of technique considers the mechanical detail of skills performed by athletes. This allows flaws in technique to be identified and changes in technique to be monitored during preparation or rehabilitation from injury. Effectiveness can be evaluated at a skill level (technical effectiveness) or more broadly looking at passages of play (effectiveness of tactics). Technical effectiveness considers the skills performed and how

6

well they have been performed according to outcome. This broadly classifies skills as being performed positively or negatively without analysing the detail of the technical movement. Technical effectiveness can be expressed in terms of the percentage of skills that are performed successfully, such as pass completion rates in team games or service rates in racket sports. For example, a player may complete 80 per cent of short passes and 64 per cent of long passes. Note, that we have not considered any detail of the passing technique when broadly looking at the effectiveness of passing. Similarly, a tennis player may win 65 per cent of service points when a flat serve is used, 60 per cent when a kick serve is used and 55 per cent when a slice serve is used. Again, no detail of the service techniques involved here has been described. The analysis of technical effectiveness can direct the use of more detailed analysis of technique (Bartlett, 2002). For example, we may decide to examine the player's kick serve which we have found to be the least productive in winning points. This involves looking at the kick serve technique in detail. The soccer example is not as straightforward as completing 64 per cent of long passes may be a better performance than completing 80 per cent of short passes. If two short passes are equivalent to a long pass, then the chance of two successive short passes being successful is 80 per cent of 80 per cent which is 64 per cent (the same chance we would have if we used a single long pass). The effectiveness of broader passages of play can also be analysed. These broad passages of play can be made up of multiple skills performed by different players. Broad possession types are deemed to be successful according to territory gained or scoring opportunities generated.

Tactical evaluation has typically used observational analysis as an indirect way of analysing tactical decisions made and broader strategies used by teams and players. By analysing patterns of events based on skills performed, locations of events, timings and the players involved, it is possible to describe tactics used. When a tennis player attacks the net, it is typically because they have made a tactical decision to do so. We make inferences about tactical decisions based on what we observe during competition. Effectiveness is typically analysed while evaluating tactics. That is, it is not just important to know what a player or team chose to do, but how well they executed the tactical choices. This allows us to compare alternative tactics in terms of their effectiveness. Consider the analysis of the Norwegian Football Squad's (1993–4) scoring opportunities from the defending half shown in Table 1.1 (Olsen and Larsen,

1997). Norway had a reputation for being a counter-attacking team who used fast direct attacks very effectively. Table 1.1 suggests that Norway's most productive attack was the one they chose to do least (build up attack). This would actually come as a surprise to scholars of Norway's soccer philosophy in the 1990s. However, the data come from a book chapter co-authored by none other than Egil Olsen, Norway's head coach at the time. It would be interesting to know the total number of each attack and not just those leading to scoring opportunities in order to understand more fully the productiveness of the different attacking styles for Norway.

Movement analysis is a term that is relevant to technique, tactics and work-rate. When analysing technique, we analyse detailed movements of joints and body segments. When analysing tactics, we analyse movements that are made by players for tactical reasons to achieve positions where they have an advantage. In time-motion analysis, movement refers to the locomotive movements performed by players and how these indicate the physical demands of the game. There are many different ways in which time-motion analysis can be done. One way is to analyse the distribution of match time among different movement classes. This can be done very broadly with just two movement classes such as work and rest (O'Donoghue *et al.*, 2005a/b), more typically with 7 to 12 movement classes (Reilly and Thomas, 1976; Withers *et al.*, 1982) or with more detailed movement classes including details of straight and arced movements, direction of movement with respect to aspect faced by the player, turns and swerves (Bloomfield *et al.*, 2004). Another way of analysing movement is to track player locations, determining velocities and the distance covered at different speed sub-ranges. This analysis of distance covered can use automatic player tracking data from GPS systems (Coutts and Duffield, 2010) or semi-automatic tracking data using image processing (Gregson *et al.*, 2010).

Table 1.1 Norway's attacks from their own defensive area in 1994

| Type of attack | Opportunity but no goal | Goal | Total | % Goals |
|---|---|---|---|---|
| Over midfield | 16 | 4 | 20 | 20.0% |
| Through midfield fast | 18 | 10 | 28 | 35.7% |
| Build up attack | 3 | 8 | 11 | 72.7% |

8

Decision making includes tactical choices made by players. The reason why O'Donoghue (2010) used a separate category for decision making was to also cover the decisions made by umpires when officiating matches. Within each of the five purposes, there are different sub-aspects and more detailed variables that can be examined. One of the key tasks in developing a sports performance analysis system is to identify the information that is needed. In this book, the terms data and information are used to represent different things. Data are input into some analysis process resulting in information being produced as an output. The selection of a relevant and important aspect of the sport to analyse is critical to the validity of any system. The analyst needs to operationalise the chosen aspect of the sport using observable and measurable characteristics of performance. Variables are devised that can be output from the system and used to support decisions. The information needed dictates the raw data that should be collected from performances and how they should be stored and processed. The process of developing an analysis system is covered in Chapter 4 including the details of how variables are defined. Later in this chapter, two examples are covered that will be used throughout the book to illustrate different aspects of sports performance analysis. These two examples give an insight into reducing the complexity of sports performance to a more abstract concise form to support decision making.

## Why do we do sports performance analysis?

Athletes and coaches make decisions about preparation that need to be informed by evidence. They need to understand areas of performance requiring attention, the tactics they can perform successfully and the strengths and weaknesses of forthcoming opponents. Sports performance analysis is used to provide coaches, high performance directors and other users with valid, accurate and reliable information about sports performances. This information helps many types of decision that coaches and athletes need to make. The use of performance analysis support helps overcome the limited recall of coaches and other observers when relying on their own observation. Coach recall was found to be limited to less than 45 per cent of critical incidents in international soccer (Franks and Miller, 1986). A more recent study of UEFA (Union of European Football Associations) pro-licence qualified coaches found that this figure has risen to 59 per cent (Laird and Waters, 2008). However, recall is still incomplete and can be inaccurate as well as open to bias and misinterpretation.

Emotion can affect assessments made from observations in general (Cohen *et al.*, 2011: 211). Performance in competitive sport is a specific example of emotion affecting the accuracy of observer perceptions. The author suggests that students experience this for themselves by attending a football match where they are also able to view recorded television coverage of the match later. At the match you should look at key refereeing decisions, whether you consider them to be correct and how supporters react to them at the time. Then look at the match recording later, specifically the incidents where you recall particular disagreements with the referee by large numbers of supporters. Was the referee's decision correct according to the rules of the game? If so, how could so many supporters have been incorrect? Were they influenced by the reaction of other supporters around them? Were they trying to pressurise the referee by displaying hostility to decisions that went against their team? Were the supporters equally vocal when a refereeing decision went against the opposing team? Was there bias involved from the supporters? If so, was this exacerbated by emotional aspects of spectating?

An example of emotional influence from the author's own experience was a boxing match he watched live at the venue where the author perceived the boxer he was supporting to be losing on points right up until the eighth round when the boxer won by way of technical knockout. Some weeks later, knowing the outcome of the bout, the author watched the full match again on video and on this occasion perceived the boxer to be comfortably ahead from the outset of the match. The television commentators, who were impartial, also considered the boxer to have been leading on points at the time he won by technical knockout.

Table 1.1 is an example of how sports performance analysis can expose misperceptions about Norway's effectiveness applying different styles of attack. Sports performance analysis provides information that overcomes such misperceptions, limitations in recall and emotional bias. It aims to be objective and is used within the feedback process to support more effective decisions.

## Who uses sports performance analysis?

Sports performance analysis is primarily used in coaching contexts to provide feedback to players helping them to direct training activity and enhance performance. Performance data can also be used by high performance directors to make decisions about funding priorities (Leyshon, 2012; Wiltshire, 2013). There are other application areas of performance analysis in sport including coach development (O'Donoghue and Mayes, 2013b). Coaches have the opportunity to have their own behaviour recorded during coaching sessions allowing them to reflect on their coaching style and identify any aspects that could be altered. A coach can be fitted with a microphone that transmits their voice to a camera which can film from a location allowing the coach to be followed without taking the camera onto the training area. Indeed, separate cameras can be used to show the wider training arena and a close up view of the coach. These two views can be provided in a split screen video that has been tagged with the coaching behaviours performed (Brown and O'Donoghue, 2008a). Such feedback to coaches can be used within a process of reflective practice during various stages of their career (Schön, 1983).

Referee performance is under scrutiny in the media and is also being monitored by sports governing bodies. The work-rate of referees (D'Ottavio and Castagna, 2001; Mizohata *et al.*, 2009) as well as the accuracy of their decisions (Rose-Doherty and O'Donoghue, 2012) have been examined in research studies. The process of refereeing or umpiring performance often involves considerable observation of the event (Mellick, 2005; Kirkbride, 2013a). The soccer referee and assistant referees observe matches live, following the action, analysing what players are doing with respect to the laws of the game (Coleclough, 2013). The judges in amateur boxing watch the contest live, using red and blue buttons to enter scoring punches they recognise during the bout (Mullan and O'Donoghue, 2001). This involves observing punches and considering these in relation to the criteria for punches to be scored in amateur boxing. Of course, soccer referees and boxing judges are not performance analysts. They are referees and judges. However, their activity undeniably involves analysing performance with an officiating or scoring purpose. They have no interest in the appropriateness of tactical decisions made by athletes, the mechanics of athletes' technique or the work-rate athletes are generating. However, they are analysing those aspects of performance that are necessary within their role. Boxing judges and judges of sports like ice-skating, gymnastics and trampolining undertake data gathering activity during performance that is similar to the data collection work typically done by performance analysts (Di Felice and Marcora, 2013; Johns and Brouner, 2013).

There are also media applications of performance analysis (James, 2008; Kirkbride, 2013b). Television channels have supplemented their coverage of sport with commentary, expert analysis during intervals and match facts which are presented in forms providing viewers with a better understanding of key aspects of matches. Match statistics provided during soccer matches include territory, possession, foul play and scoring opportunity statistics. In sports such as tennis, the match statistics include serve direction breakdown shown on court diagrams, pie charts of different point types and bar charts or tables showing the proportion of different point types won by the players contesting a match.

**Where is sports performance analysis done?**

Sports performance analysis consists of a number of phases; data gathering, analysis of data and communication of information to coaches and players. These tasks can be done in various locations. Data gathering does not just include the capture of match video, but also involves the recording of skills performed by the athletes (Hughes, 2008; O'Donoghue, 2013a). The author of this book has worked in performance analysis since 1994 and has gathered data in the following locations:

- At match venues (indoors and outdoors).
- At home (when matches are being shown live or replayed later on television).
- At home when analysing a recorded match video recorded.
- On buses, aircraft and trains as well as airport departure lounges when travelling home from matches.
- In hotel rooms when on tour with a squad.
- In fully equipped performance analysis laboratories.
- In his office at the university.

Once the data are entered into performance analysis systems, they can also be analysed at the locations listed above. This author has certainly analysed sports performance data at all of the locations listed above.

Internet technology now permits analysts to support touring squads without having to tour with the athletes. The analyst can work remotely analysing broadcast coverage, emailing analysis reports and using an electronic drop box to provide supporting video clips.

# 12

Communication of information to players needs to be done with extra care to ensure the feedback is effective. Players need to be comfortable with the environment in which they are receiving feedback especially if the feedback may be critical of aspects of their play. Match briefings and debriefings can be done in meeting rooms that are organised for this purpose or within performance analysis laboratories that are equipped for such presentations and related interaction between coaches and players. Hotel rooms have also been used on tour to allow units within teams to view feedback and discuss performance when on tour. Some players also use travel time to view video sequences that have been identified as a result of performance analysis. Changing rooms are an additional location of motivational feedback in the author's experience.

## When is sports performance analysis done?

When you ask practising sports performance analysts to describe their work between and during matches, they typically advise that the same process does not occur in each match to match cycle. There may be different information needs and areas to focus on when preparing for one match than another. However, there are general processes that are frequently used with some variation in the tasks to be done. Once a system is developed and is in operation, sports performance analysis involves the stages of data gathering, analysis and communication of information to coaches and players. These stages can be performed at different times with respect to the time at which the match is played depending on the purpose of the analysis. Broadly speaking, sports performance analysis can be classified into real-time analysis and post-match analysis.

Real-time analysis is where data are entered while the competition is taking place and analysis allows information to be communicated to coaches and players during competition. The statistics window of sportscode (O'Donoghue, 2013a) allows executable scripts to process data entered by users and sent to output windows that can appear on wireless devices in the possession of coaches. For example, such a system can be used with the analyst working from a good camera viewing location while the coach receives live match statistics during the match on an iPad or iPhone device. The technology available today also allows athletes on substitute benches to see delayed video feeds of game action.

This can help understand the way opponents play before the substitutes are introduced to the match.

There are many other examples of live feedback being provided to performers in the competition arena. One only has to look at the coverage of Formula One motor racing to see the extent of data used to make decisions during competition. At a more basic level, mere mortals like the author get feedback when exercising in his local gym. The author was also recently video recorded by a friend's mobile phone while exercising on a rowing machine. This allowed discussion of flawed technique and how technique might be improved.

Post-match analysis is where data are analysed and information communicated to players after the match. The additional time allows for more detailed analysis than is possible with real-time analysis. Some systems combined real-time analysis and post-match analysis. They gather some critically important data during competition with other more detailed data being compiled after the match. The times at which data are gathered and analysed are usually dictated by the purpose for which the data are to be used.

When we consider the different application contexts of sports performance analysis, there are many different analyses that are required and they may be required at different times. For example, in a coaching context, information may be required for a debriefing session before the next match or before the next training session. More in-depth analysis involving multiple match data may be required before the next match against a particular opponent. Continuous monitoring of players, teams and opponents continues with databases being populated so that information can be retrieved when it is required.

The media application area is an interesting one to discuss because the timescales involved give an indication of the technological and manpower resources required. Television coverage of matches requires statistical information and supporting video sequences to be available for the half time interval and shortly after the match has finished. Consider the end sequence of a television programme where highlights of the match are shown accompanied by music and credits. This is close to the task of producing a motivational video but needs to be ready within an hour of the match finishing. A media technician is probably gathering candidate clips during the match and has a shortlist of three or four pieces of music of the required duration to be used. The credits may be

14

standard with some specific acknowledgements to include and can be set up before the match begins. The video may commence with an early video clip of the teams walking onto the pitch which gives the technician a good start to producing the video.

Analysis for print media will have strict deadlines for material to be included in certain editions. Columns of newspapers will have already been reserved for reports, images and related analyses from the known fixtures taking place on the day. The reporters might not analyse the match quantitatively themselves but may draw on publicly available match statistics or subcontract the sports performance analysis task to commercial providers of such information such as Opta™ (www.optasports.com).

Match statistics are provided on the official websites of professional clubs as well as the official websites of tournaments. These statistics are often provided while matches are still in progress and can be used by television channels, newspapers and private individuals. IBM presents statistics on tennis matches at Grand Slam tournaments. Tennis is an ideal sport for such analysis as there is a 20s interval between points within games and longer intervals between games and sets. The analysts working at Grand Slam tournaments can enter point details on palm top devices while they watch the matches. Recently, businesses have been created that provide such data for the purposes of 'infotainment' (Kirkbride, 2013b). Customers can access this information on mobile phones, tablets and other devices. Some may use the information out of personal interest while others may use the information to make decisions about bets to be made on matches. Betting agencies now provide internet sites and access from mobile devices permitting bets to be made live during matches. This has fostered a market for live sports performance data and provided further employment for analysts.

The reliability of the data provided on websites should be independently verified before using the data for any serious purpose. The definitions of variables may be vague. The variables may be defined in training courses for the analysts who will collect data but are not provided publicly to the consumers of the resulting information.

The times at which academic performance analysis activities are done also depends on their purpose. Typically, results are not required immediately after matches. Instead, matches may be recorded and analysed with further reductive analysis done to provide average match results. The analysis needs to be done in sufficient time to permit academic reports to be written up for module deadlines. This applies to formal coursework as well as independent research projects. Students may do practical exercises during modules that more realistically reflect the nature of sports performance analysis in professional contexts. Scope for doing this may be limited because the students are not full-time analysts and do have other modules to work for within their programmes of study.

Research active university academics do research to be presented at conferences or published in academic journals. Where a study is to be presented at a conference, the analysis must be done permitting a summary abstract of the research including its main findings to be submitted before the deadline set by the scientific committee of the conference. Further detailed analysis, the production of slides and/or posters can be done prior to the conference. Some conferences, such as the Science and Football Conferences, produce proceedings that are published as books (Nunome *et al.*, 2013). The World Congress of Performance Analysis of Sport has been held nine times between 1992 and 2012, with the proceedings of the most recent congress being published as a book of 41 chapters (Peters and O'Donoghue, 2013). There will be set deadlines for chapters to be completed by authors to be included in such proceedings. Other conferences produce books of proceedings available for delegates attending the conference. This requires much tighter deadlines for authors than when proceedings are being produced after the event. Publishing in academic journals does not involve such tight deadlines because where authors fail to submit a paper in time for it to be reviewed, revised and edited for one issue of the journal, there will be future issues of the journal that the paper could be published in.

The examples above have been concerned with situations where a stable analysis process exists with standard information requirements and data sources. However, most practising analysts are continually developing and modifying systems to meet changing requirements from coaches and other customers. Minor modifications to systems can be done as and when information requirements change. More extensive changes to systems may be restricted to the months between seasons for the particular sport the analyst is involved in. Commercial organisations that provide sports performance analysis services to professional soccer clubs have a very small amount of time between one season ending and another commencing to engage in product development activity. The preliminary rounds of European club tournaments, for example, start shortly after major international tournaments finish.

16

## How is sports performance analysis done? The methods

In answering the question 'How do we do sports performance analysis?' we are considering the methods that are used. The sports performance analysis community has grown over the last 30 years and, as it has done so, the methods adopted have also expanded. In the 1980s, the term sports performance analysis was not really used by the community and methods were largely restricted to notational analysis methods. Even with the advent of computerised systems, replacing shorthand notation with function keys and on-screen buttons of graphical user interfaces (GUIs), the term 'computerised notation' was used. Indeed, the professional body of the area was the International Society of Notational Analysis of Sport with the first three World Congresses of the society being entitled World Congress of Notational Analysis (Buron Manor, 1992, Liverpool 1994 and Antalya, 1996). It was Keith Lyons who proposed that the area would be better termed 'performance analysis' in his keynote address at the Fourth World Congress in Porto in 1998. This keynote address also proposed that performance analysis was at the centre of sports science and not on the periphery. Book chapters by Hughes and Bartlett (2004 and 2008) described performance analysis as comprising biomechanics and notational analysis. O'Donoghue (2010) proposed a more expansive array of methods that could be covered by sports performance analysis. The term 'sports performance analysis' started to be used instead of 'performance analysis' around 2010 in recognition that performance analysis is done in many fields of work, not just sport. As has already been discussed earlier in this chapter, sports performance analysis is the analysis of actual sports performance although there is a role for laboratory studies to analyse important skills that cannot be analysed in the competition scenario. Qualitative observational methods are used and these pre-date the work of the notational analysis community. More objective and quantitative methods are also used. Computerised match analysis with integrated video is now commonplace, but there is still a role for manual notation methods, especially where filming is not permitted. The scope of this book does not include detailed analysis of technique which will be covered by another book in the series. The main methods that will be covered in the book are manual notational analysis (Chapter 5 and 6), computerised match analysis (Chapters 7 and 8) and computerised time-motion analysis (Chapters 7, 8 and 9).

## TWO PURPOSES OF SPORTS PERFORMANCE ANALYSIS

### Match analysis

The main application areas of sports performance analysis and its main purposes have been discussed earlier in this chapter. The current section of the chapter provides greater detail about two broad purposes of sports performance analysis with the aid of examples that will be used throughout the book. The first of these two purposes is match analysis and this will be illustrated using the example of serving strategy in tennis. Match analysis is used to analyse game sports and involves data about individual skills. For example, data from a soccer match may be recorded for each event that occurred; the skill type (pass, shot, tackle, etc.), the team that performed the skill, the player that performed the skill, the pitch location of the skill (the pitch may be divided into nine areas for the purpose of analysis), the time at which the skill was performed and the outcome of the skill (successful or unsuccessful execution). These data can be analysed to show how well the teams and individual players executed different types of skill. This type of analysis can also be done with respect to periods of the match and locations of the pitch. This is an example of technical effectiveness because the success with which skills are performed is analysed while detail of the techniques used is not addressed. These data could also be used for tactical analysis; if a team decides to play more on the left and right wings than other teams, the event frequencies will reflect this tactical choice made by the team. The specific example used here is tennis serving and Table 1.2 is an example of the results that can be produced for a match. The match in question is the 2012 US Open men's singles final between Andy Murray and Novak Djokovic.

Table 1.2 represents all points except double faults. The following data were recorded for each point:

- The serving player
- Whether the point emanated from a first or second serve
- Whether the serving player was serving to the deuce or advantage court
- The third of the target service box where the serve landed if it was in
- Whether or not the serving player won the point

18

**Table 1.2** Proportion of points won serving to different areas of the service courts in the 2012 US Open Men's singles final (Won/Played) (www.usopen.org, accessed 31 December 2012)

| | Deuce court | | | Advantage court | | |
| | Left | Middle | Right | Left | Middle | Right |
|---|---|---|---|---|---|---|
| *Andy Murray* | | | | | | |
| 1st serve | 20/28 | 4/13 | 7/7 | 11/22 | 9/14 | 10/14 |
| 2nd serve | 0/1 | 15/28 | 1/2 | 0/1 | 8/14 | 1/2 |
| | | | | | | |
| *Novak Djokovic* | | | | | | |
| 1st serve | 11/20 | 8/14 | 15/21 | 11/19 | 8/11 | 15/18 |
| 2nd serve | 4/7 | 9/19 | 0/1 | 1/4 | 11/24 | 1/2 |

This simple analysis does not include information about groundstrokes or volleys played within the point, whether either player went to the net or whether the point was won with a winner or an opponent error and if any errors were forced or unforced. However, this simple analysis can still give an insight into the performance of the two players which might support decisions about preparation for future matches. Consider Andy Murray's first serve performance; he tended to serve more to the left (Djokovic's forehand) than to the right when serving to both deuce and advantage courts. However, Andy Murray was more successful when serving to the right so we may ask the question 'Why did he not serve to the right more often?' Novak Djokovic served a similar number of points to the left and the right when serving to deuce and advantage courts. However, like Murray, Djokovic was more successful when serving to the right (the opponent's backhand side) so we can speculate whether he should have served there more frequently. Those inspecting the results in Table 1.2 may conclude that rather than serving more often to the right, the players need to be more productive when serving to the left. This allows coaches and players to focus on relevant video sequences to identify how productivity can be improved when serving to the left. Both players adopted a similar strategy of serving to the middle third of the target service box more often than not on second serve. We could use percentages in Table 1.2 along with the frequencies; for example 1/4 = 25 per cent. This is fine as long as we are aware that, if one of the three lost points had been won, the percentage would be 50 per cent. Sometimes, percentages can be judged inappropriately when there are low event frequencies. This example of tennis serving will be used as an example in Chapters 6 and 8 and will have an additional variable incorporated which is the type of serve used. Serve type is classified as flat, kick or slice.

**Work-rate analysis**

Work-rate analysis is the analysis of the physical demands of a sport through observational means. This area has a number of different names including work-rate analysis, time-motion analysis and movement analysis. There have been reviews of work-rate analysis published in journals and books in recent years. The main secondary sources of material on research in this area are the reviews of Carling and Bloomfield (2013), Carling *et al.* (2008) and O'Donoghue (2008a). There are many different ways of undertaking work-rate analysis using different methods that exploit a range of technologies. Since the earliest days of work-rate analysis in sport, there have been methods based on distances covered and other methods where the distribution of time among named movements is determined (Reilly and Thomas, 1976; Withers *et al.*, 1982). The methods based on distance covered have benefited from advances in player tracking technology (Carling *et al.*, 2008). Player tracking systems based on radio signals, GPS equipment and image processing determine the location of players periodically throughout matches or training sessions. For example, the Prozone3 player tracking system (Prozone Sports Ltd, Leeds, UK) records the X,Y co-ordinates of all players on the field 10 times per second (10 Hz). These data are then manually verified by quality assurance personnel before the data are available to the clubs who use them. The manual verification process and other measurement information relating to Prozone3 are described by Di Salvo *et al.* (2009). The timed X,Y co-ordinates (referred to as player trajectories) allow a variety of outputs to be determined through simple processing. Applying Pythagoras theory to the data allows distances covered to be estimated. The author uses the word 'estimated' because even if the X,Y co-ordinates are accurate to the nearest mm, the players would not have always moved the shortest straight line between a pair of locations separated by a 0.1s interval. Given that the distances covered are estimated every 0.1s, movement speeds can also be determined by dividing distances over known times. Similarly, accelerations can be estimated given that initial and final speeds are estimated for given time periods. Typically, accelerations would be produced using 0.5s data rather than every 0.1s. This is necessary to avoid the propagation of error in individual 0.1s intervals.

20

If there is an average inaccuracy of 0.2m (for example) in the location recorded at any point in time, there is a potential inaccuracy of 0.4m in the distance calculated for a 0.1s period. This is because the error at the start of the interval could be in the opposite direction to the error at the end of the interval. Where we have a time period of 0.5s, this potential error of 0.4s is smaller in relative terms to the distance covered than it would be if we were considering a time period of 0.1s. The total distance travelled in different speed ranges during the match can be determined as well as the frequency and durations of periods spent moving in those speed ranges. For example, the frequency and duration of high speed running (defined by Di Salvo $et$ $al.$ (2009) as being performed at 19.8 km.hour$^{-1}$ (5.5m.s$^{-1}$) or faster) has received attention in research and provides information to coaches about the intermittent nature of players' high speed running. Some use universal speed thresholds for different movements while others prefer player specific speed thresholds. The Prozone3 system can be tailored to provide information using speed thresholds that recognise the different sprinting abilities of players. More complex algorithms have been written to analyse player trajectories, recognising the times at which players perform cutting movements (O'Donoghue and Robinson, 2009). Indeed, the possibilities are endless and just require the system development effort to realise any output that can be feasibly determined from player trajectory data.

The other class of work-rate analysis methods is based on the classification of movement by human observers. The number of different movements in classification schemes ranges from 2 to over 80. The POWER (Periods Of Work Effort and Recoveries) system uses two broad movement classes, 'work' and 'rest' (O'Donoghue $et$ $al.$, 2005a). Others have used 7 to 12 movement classes to cover different types of work and rest activity that are of interest (Bangsbo $et$ $al.$, 1991; Huey $et$ $al.$, 2001). These include rest activities such as standing, walking forwards, walking backwards or sideways and jogging as well as work activities such as running, sprinting, on-the-ball activity and high intensity shuffling movements. The most complex movement classification scheme was developed by Bloomfield to investigate the agility requirements of soccer (Bloomfield $et$ $al.$, 2004). Bloomfield realised that the traditional methods of work-rate analysis did not provide any information about accelerations, decelerations, changes of direction, cross-over runs, or whether different movements were performed moving forwards, backwards, sideways or in arced directions. Furthermore, speed agility quickness training was being done by professional players without there being any scientific understanding of the agility requirements of different sports. Bloomfield's movement classification addressed this and has been used to understand the demands of soccer (Bloomfield *et al.*, 2007) and netball (Williams and O'Donoghue, 2005).

Within the current text book, work-rate analysis is used as an example of computerised performance analysis as well as an example of reliability. Therefore, in this introductory chapter, the typical human operated movement classification schemes will be described. We will use a two movement scheme (work and rest) and a seven movement scheme (stationary, walking, backing, jogging, running/sprinting, shuffling, on-the-ball). This may seem like a step back in time given the existence of sophisticated player tracking systems. However, player tracking technology is not available to all universities and the human observer alternative is a good educational example of measurement issues relevant to sports performance analysis. Huey *et al.* (2001) provided some definitions for the movements in the seven movement scheme; these are listed in Chapter 9. The definitions offer some guidance to operators. However, attempting to produce operational definitions can be counter-productive as we will discuss in Chapter 2 and Chapter 9.

The frequency, mean duration and percentage match time spent performing these movements can be presented in a table such as Table 1.3 or a pie chart could be used to show the distribution of match time. The software used to record movement instances can also be programmed to string together consecutively performed low intensity activities (stationary, walking, backing and jogging) as well as consecutively performed high intensity activities (running, shuffling and game-related activity). This allows broad periods of high intensity activity and low intensity activity to be identified. As shown in Table 1.3, the frequency, mean duration and percentage match time spent performing low and high intensity activity can be output. One would expect high and low intensity activities to alternate and, therefore, expect the number of high and low intensity periods to differ by no more than one. In soccer, there are two halves in a match and so we can sometimes observe a difference of two between these frequencies.

Table 1.3 can be used to determine that the total playing time was 96 mins 25.5s (950 movements × 6.09 s mean duration). We can also see that soccer involves intermittent high intensity activity with the particular

Table 1.3 Frequency, mean duration and percentage time a soccer player spent performing different locomotive movements

| Activity | Frequency | Mean duration (s) | %Time |
|---|---|---|---|
| Stationary | 98 | 6.58 | 11.14 |
| Walking | 326 | 9.98 | 56.21 |
| Backing | 156 | 4.28 | 11.53 |
| Jogging | 217 | 4.13 | 15.47 |
| Running | 47 | 2.35 | 1.91 |
| Shuffling | 76 | 1.91 | 2.51 |
| Game-related activity | 30 | 2.53 | 1.22 |
| Total | 950 | 6.09 | 100.00 |
| High intensity activity | 124 | 2.63 | 5.64 |
| Low intensity activity | 126 | 43.34 | 94.36 |

player performing 124 bursts of high intensity activity of average duration 2.63s. The player is involved in on-the-ball activity or challenging for the ball for 1.22 per cent of the match which seems low. However, when one considers that 55 minutes of a 90 minute soccer match is live ball-in-play time (O'Donoghue and Parker, 2001), that this 55 minutes is shared between 22 players, and that the ball will be travelling between players for some of the time, some players will spend less than two minutes in game-related activity. The modal movement is walking forwards; indeed this player spent more time walking forwards than he spent performing all the other activities added together.

If we are primarily concerned with work and rest and not the different types of work and rest movements, then a two movement classification system could be used to record 'work' and 'rest' respectively. This is an unashamedly subjective system where the operator enters work where they perceive the player under observation to be performing high intensity activity. Rest is entered for any other activity that is perceived to be performed at a low or moderate intensity. Applying this system to the same player analysed using the seven movement classification scheme gave the output shown in Table 1.4.

The durations in Table 1.4 are means for the whole performance but not all periods of work (or rest) are of the mean duration for work (or rest). Therefore, the POWER system also shows the number of work and rest periods of different durations. These can be cross-tabulated, as in Table 1.5, so that we can see the durations of rest periods that follow short,

Table 1.4 Frequency, mean duration and percentage time a soccer player spent performing work and rest

|  | Frequency | Mean duration (s) | %Time |
|---|---|---|---|
| *First half* | | | |
| Rest | 70 | 37.83 | 91.58 |
| Work | 69 | 3.53 | 8.42 |
| *Second half* | | | |
| Rest | 73 | 36.14 | 90.50 |
| Work | 72 | 3.85 | 9.50 |
| *Match* | | | |
| Rest | 143 | 36.97 | 91.04 |
| Work | 141 | 3.69 | 8.96 |

medium and long periods of work. The total column on the right of Table 1.5 shows that 115 of the 141 work periods (81.6 per cent) lasted less than six seconds. The mean recovery might be 36.97s, but only 52 of the 114 recoveries (36.9 per cent of them) were in the median rest duration banding of 20–45s. There were 35 (24.8 per cent) rest periods of less than eight seconds meaning that there were occasions where the player performed work without having a full recovery from the previous work effort. Hence, some work-rate analysis studies have used the concept of repeated work (or sprint) bouts (Spencer *et al.*, 2004; O'Donoghue *et al.*, 2005b). The two and seven movement classification schemes will be used in Chapter 9 to illustrate computerised systems and reliability assessment.

Table 1.5 Number of work periods of different durations followed by rest periods of different durations by the soccer player

| Work duration | Recovery duration | | | | | | | | |
|---|---|---|---|---|---|---|---|---|---|
| | 0–2s | 2–4s | 4–8s | 8–12s | 12–20s | 20–45s | 45–90s | 90s+ | Total |
| 0–2s | 4 | 1 | 8 | 0 | 10 | 9 | 5 | 2 | 39 |
| 2–4s | 4 | 5 | 3 | 1 | 2 | 16 | 11 | 7 | 49 |
| 4–6s | 3 | 0 | 0 | 0 | 1 | 15 | 4 | 4 | 27 |
| 6–8s | 1 | 3 | 1 | 3 | 2 | 6 | 1 | 1 | 18 |
| 8–10s | 1 | 0 | 0 | 0 | 0 | 0 | 2 | 2 | 5 |
| 10–12s | 0 | 0 | 0 | 0 | 0 | 2 | 0 | 0 | 2 |
| 12s+ | 0 | 0 | 1 | 0 | 0 | 0 | 0 | 0 | 1 |
| Total | 13 | 9 | 13 | 4 | 15 | 48 | 23 | 16 | 141 |

24

## SUMMARY

Sports performance analysis is the analysis of actual sports performance. There is a wide variety of methods that can be used within the scope of sports performance analysis ranging from highly qualitative methods to highly quantitative methods with little or no human judgement during data collection. There are times when we need to analyse technique in detail but can only do so within a laboratory setting. Where such laboratory studies are analysing key skills of the sport, they fall within the scope of sports performance analysis. There are coaching, media, judging and academic application contexts of sports performance analysis. The main purposes of sports performance analysis are analysis of technique, tactical analysis and work-rate analysis. Analysis is not limited to players and teams because coach behaviour and referee performance can also be analysed. The main rationale for sports performance analysis is that it helps overcome the limitations of observer recall. The information gathered is typically more objective and complete and can support decision making by coaches and players.

# CHAPTER 2

## QUANTITATIVE AND QUALITATIVE ANALYSIS

### INTRODUCTION

The traditional rationale for performance analysis has highlighted limited recall ability of coaches as well as potentially biased and inaccurate recollection of match events (Franks and Miller, 1986; 1991; Laird and Waters, 2008). However, subjective observation, which is often used by coaches, also has advantages over the more objective quantitative methods. This chapter describes the use of qualitative and quantitative analysis when applied within sports performance analysis, discussing their relative strengths and weaknesses.

Table 2.1 lists the key differences between qualitative and quantitative techniques. Qualitative data are typically complex and include visual patterns, video, words, feelings, thoughts and emotions. The meanings of such data are interpreted by those analysing them and typically rely on personal judgement. Quantitative data are typically facts and figures that are not open to personal interpretation but are analysed using

Table 2.1 Differences between qualitative and quantitative methods

| Qualitative | Quantitative |
| --- | --- |
| Subjective | Objective |
| Matter of opinion | Matter of fact |
| Judgement | Measurement |
| Applying experience, expertise | Following detailed guidance |
| Interpretation | Statistical analysis |
| Flexible process | Fixed process |

26

statistical methods. Another way of thinking about the difference between quantitative and qualitative techniques is to think of the words 'quantity' and 'quality'. Quantitative methods can be used to count the number of passes made in a game, the number of passes that reach a team mate, and convert these into a percentage of passes played that reach a team mate. There is a lot of information lost when passes are simply classified by outcome. However, this approach can be used to manage complex performance data, reducing it to a manageable form supporting decision making. Qualitative methods, on the other hand, can be used to consider the quality of passing technique used. In other words, a pass is not just counted as having occurred and having been successful or not.

This chapter discusses different types of data and how they are analysed. First, qualitative methods are discussed before three further sections introduce quantitative methods. It is important to distinguish between truly objective measures with no human judgement and those methods that have traditionally been considered as objective despite involving subjective classification processes by human observers. The second section covers methods where there is no human judgement during data collection. These involve automated systems such as Hawkeye (Hawkeye Innovations, Basingstoke, UK) and some player tracking technologies. The third section covers traditional notational analysis techniques where human observers classify behaviour, counting or timing events that are performed. While the results of such analyses appear to be quantitative and presented as charts or tables of numeric values, the raw data are subjective at the point of data collection. The fourth section of the chapter covers performance analysis techniques involving human observers without the need for observers to subjectively classify behaviour. These methods involve decisions by persons other than the analysts. For example, in tennis we could analyse point outcomes according to umpire decisions, removing the need for analysts to judge whether balls are played in or out of court.

## QUALITATIVE DATA AND ANALYSIS

### Qualitative observation

There is a wide range of qualitative methods used in sports science research including ethnography, auto-ethnography, accounts, interviews, focus groups and observation. Non-participant observation is the method of most relevance to sports performance analysis. Participant observation is where the researcher engages in the activity being studied in order to experience the activity and the wider culture that it takes place in. The term 'researcher' is being used very broadly here to cover a full range of application areas including coaching, academic research, police work and journalism. There are ethical concerns with methods where researchers covertly investigate groups using deception to gain access and effectively infiltrate the group. Non-participant observation, on the other hand, is where the researcher investigates the behaviour of interest without personally engaging in it. This is typically done overtly with groups under observation being aware of the researcher's role. The coach, observing athletes training without the aid of a performance analyst, will be doing so with the athletes' full knowledge of this. Players competing in sports events that are televised or displayed on other media channels will be aware that their performances can be evaluated by viewers.

Qualitative methods have been used in coaching and predate the use of notational analysis (Hayes, 1997). Coaches typically observe performance during training and competition, evaluating athlete performance based on knowledge of the sport. During training, the coach has the option to intervene and provide feedback periodically. Other possibilities for the coach during training are to analyse the activities of athletes specifically to help confirm areas of performance requiring attention. During competition, there is less scope for intervention and providing feedback, even in sports with half and quarter time intervals and time-outs.

Sports performance analysis has been portrayed as an objective means of providing accurate information to coaches and players. However, there are sports performance analysis tasks that are more subjective in nature where analysts exercise judgement during observation. The author once worked with a squad where a completely subjective system was applied during the preparation for a major championship. There were other more objective systems that the author was using routinely with the squad at this time, but there was a need for the subjective system during squad training. The goal of the subjective system was to provide players with highlight videos of their involvement in training games. The author filmed the training games entering events that could potentially be used in feedback videos for players. For each event, the author had to press two buttons on the computerised system. One button was either 'Positive' or 'Negative' depending on the quality of the player's involvement in the

28

event. The second button identified the player performing the event. There was a choice of 18 such buttons because there were 18 players in the squad at that time.

The events recorded were relative to different players' abilities. For example, there were events that might be recorded as a positive event for some players that would not be recorded as such for the higher ability players in the squad. This was because these events would be considered typical and expected for the higher ability players. So the positive events that were recorded were events that would be considered positive and worthy of feeding back relative to the ability of the player. Similarly, there were events that might be recorded as negative for the high ability players that would not be recorded as such for other players in the squad. This was because the events might be performed in difficult circumstances and a negative outcome might be understandable for some players in the squad but not for the higher ability players. Relating the quality of execution of an event to player ability meant that a similar volume of events could be fed back to each player. Each player would see events considered to be positive and negative given their current ability.

The author was also able to take into account more complex factors by having the freedom to subjectively classify events as positive or negative. Such factors included the degree of difficulty of the event, the degree of success of the event, appropriateness of decision making, quality of immediate opposition and quality of team-mates. Some events are more difficult to perform than others; for example not all backhand ground strokes in tennis are the same. When we consider placement, pace and spin of the incoming ball to be played on the backhand side, there are differences between backhand strokes which are not recorded by many objective approaches. An unrestricted subjective analysis gives the analyst freedom to consider such factors. The quality of execution of an event is rarely a black and white issue. Consider the soccer defender wishing to reach a ball on the wing of the defensive third of the field and play the ball up field. An opposing striker also wishes to reach the ball and play a cross into the penalty area. As the players reach the ball, the ball is played by the defender, striking the opposing striker's leg and goes off field for a throw in to the defender's team. Neither player achieved their objective but some systems force the analyst to record such a one-on-one duel as being won by one player or the other (Gerisch and Reicheldt, 1991). A subjective approach permits the analyst to take into account the extent to which each player achieved their goal. Very often, in performance analysis, we record what players do without recording other options that could have been taken. The events performed may be considered as matter of fact. However, the alternative options available to a player are not so straightforward and require knowledgeable analysts to be able to consider these. Subjective approaches allow the analyst to consider whether the option chosen was a good choice or not irrespective of how well the event was performed. Consider the situation where a soccer player takes a shot without a preceding touch to control the ball. The shot may miss the goal, but if the player had taken an extra touch, the opposing defence would have had enough time to prevent a shot from being taken. Therefore, despite the negative execution of the shot, the analyst can take into consideration that taking the shot was the best tactical option in the given situation. The quality of opposition has an influence on event execution. A rebound attempt in netball may be considered differently if a player is challenged for the rebound by a higher or lower ability opponent. Similarly, passages of defensive play can be considered differently depending on the players involved. In netball or basketball, a team defends for a period of time where the opposing team has the ball. This is not an instantaneous event like a pass or a tackle, but a period of opposition offense where the team's defence is evaluated. In netball, the quality of defending of a circle defender can be assessed considering the team mate who is also playing as a circle defender. In basketball, the quality of defending can consider the five players on court. What may be considered as relatively typical defending with a high quality partner(s) in defence might be considered good quality defending with a lesser ability defensive partner.

The subjective approach described here also allows events to be attributed to more than one player. For example, positive or negative defending might be attributed to two or more players within a team. An incomplete pass may be considered as negative play by both the passer and the intended receiver. The subjective approach allows the analyst to make such decisions based on knowledge and the audio-visual information that is available. While this approach is useful for rapidly producing feedback videos that are relative to player abilities, there are limitations that need to be considered. The positive to negative ratios produced this way should not be used for selection purposes. They are relative positive to relative negative ratios and players are not being compared using the same criteria for identifying positive and negative events.

30

## Photographs

While live observation and post-match video observation have been the main source of raw data used in sports performance analysis, other work has used photographic images or single video frames in the analysis of important aspects of performance. The work of Lafont (2007, 2008) on the head position in tennis during the hitting phase of shots is a good illustration of this. The qualitative analysis of photographic images revealed differences between elite players and other professional players with elite players' head position showing fixation in the direction of the contact zone at impact and during follow through. Related to the analysis of photographs is the analysis of single frames of video. We often see video sequences paused during analysis within television coverage to allow tactical aspects to be discussed and options highlighted.

## The 'inner athlete'

In addition to qualitative analysis during observational activities, qualitative methods have also been done to study the experience of performance. Specifically, 'self-confrontation' interviews (Theureau, 2003) have been used to study unobservable aspects of performance such as emotions, thoughts and feelings of the athlete during the performance (Poziat *et al.*, 2013). This type of interview is conducted while showing the athlete video sequences from their performance and asking them to discuss their experience of the performance 'from the inside'. This provides information about actual sports performance that could not be gathered using purely observational means.

## Qualitative movement diagnosis

Consider a 400m track athlete doing a training session of 200m repetitions. As the athlete runs the bend and then covers the straight to the finish line, two club coaches watch, not talking, just watching, engrossed in the observation, taking in as much information as they can. One stops the stopwatch as the athlete crosses the line but only then looks away from the athlete to check the time after the athlete has decelerated at the end of the run. The coaches briefly discuss aspects of the athlete's technique and agree what they will advise the athlete before the next repetition is performed. The athlete reaches the two coaches while walking around the track towards the 200m start line. The coaches give brief feedback walking part of the way with the athlete. This is an example of 'qualitative movement diagnosis' (Knudson, 2013). Qualitative movement diagnosis is made up of four phases (Knudson, 2013: 1):

- Preparation
- Observation
- Evaluation and Diagnosis
- Intervention

Preparation involves developing knowledge necessary to observe, evaluate and intervene. The analyst needs knowledge of the event, how the event is won or high scores obtained and the aspects of the event that are associated with success. Knowledge about the event can come from direct personal experience, professional development courses and education. The knowledge of the event includes knowledge of the critical features of the event, the temporal structure of the event, relationships between different aspects of the event and abilities required for different tasks. Knowledge of events includes models of the end result of performance in terms of other aspects of the performance. For example, Hay and Reid (1988) used a hierarchical model of the long jump to show how different aspects contributed to the distance achieved. Knowledge of common faults made in an event and how to look for these help make the observer a more informed analyst.

It is also important to have knowledge about the performer. Not all athletes are the same and their individual anthropometric characteristics, attentional style, other psychological factors, physical ability and experience may all require them to perform differently from others in the same event (Knudson, 2013: 86–7).

Observation is best done when being properly prepared to observe. Understanding the nature of the event can allow an abstract conceptual model to be used as a guide. The observation process involves the use of senses and perception as well as knowledge of skills. Data collection forms can be designed cross-tabulating body component with temporal phases of the event (Gangstead and Beveridge, 1984). These allow notes to be recorded in a systematic way.

When using qualitative methods to assess technique, observation strategies should consider the number of repetitions of an event that need to be done. The causes of performance errors may be far removed from the effects of those errors (Knudson, 2013: vii) and it may require repeated observation to identify these causes.

Evaluation and diagnosis considers a range of critical features, prioritising them according to their impact on overall performance and whether they can be corrected in the short term or long term. The evaluation compares the observed performance with an ideal performance (Knudson, 2013: 117).

The intervention stage of Knudson's (2013) approach involves providing feedback to athletes. Knudson (2013: 138) advised keeping feedback specific, positive, using a variety of approaches. For a more in-depth coverage of 'qualitative movement diagnosis', the author recommends Knudson's (2013) book on the subject which has been referred to on several occasions in the current section.

## Technological aids in qualitative analysis

The previous subsections have briefly discussed the use of qualitative observation by coaches and analysts. The use of qualitative methods does not rule out the use of technology and the purpose of the current subsection of this chapter is to discuss examples of technology being used to support qualitative approaches. This is an area that is developing rapidly; during the week when the chapter was drafted, the author was working one day in the performance analysis laboratory at Cardiff Metropolitan University which overlooks the university's outdoor 400m athletics track. An athlete and a colleague had set up a series of hurdles. The colleague used the video camera option on an iPad and filmed the athlete completing a run successfully negotiating the hurdles. The athlete walked back at the end of the run and they both viewed the clip that had been recorded. There were no numerical values, just the video containing rich complex information that could be analysed without the constraints of a narrower quantitative analysis.

In the 2009 Carling Cup final, Manchester Utd beat Tottenham Hotspur 4–1 on penalties after the match ended 0–0 after extra time. The *Guardian* described how Manchester Utd's goal keeping coach, Eric Steele, used an iPod to help goalkeeper, Ben Foster, prepare for the penalty shootout (www.guardian.co.uk/sport/blog/2009/mar/02/manchester-united-carlingcup accessed 2 July 2013). Ben Foster watched videos of his opponents taking penalty kicks on the iPod while on the pitch during the short break between extra time and the penalty shootout. The *Sun* also covered this story (www.thesun.co.uk/sol/homepage/sport/ football/2283950/Ben-Foster-became-Man-Utds-Carling-Cup-final-hero-thanks-to-his-i-Pod.html accessed 2 July 2013) including the following quote from Ben Foster:

> Just before the shootout I was looking at an iPod with goalkeeping coach Eric Steele. On it were images of Spurs taking penalties ...I'd been told if O'Hara took a kick that he would probably go to my left. It was great, that was exactly what happened and I managed to get a hand to it...I did an awful lot of research on who takes penalties for Spurs...I'd been given a lot of information on which way they put kicks...the iPod is Eric's innovation. It's an amazing tool, you can brush up straight away.

In some sports, coaches can have a screen available to them on the sideline providing a delayed feed of the match video. Action can be so fast that it is not always possible to identify everything that has happened live. While a delayed feed of a match video may not show slow motion replays or replays from multiple action, it can still assist the coach identify more about what has happened than was achieved during the live viewing of the action. The original viewing of the action allows the coach to understand the situation that has occurred, the possible outcomes and what the referee has decided. The coach can then watch the delayed feed of the incident (say ten seconds later) specifically focusing on the information needed to verify whether the referee's decision was correct or not. This principle of using the original live view and then a more focused observation of the delayed feed also applies to player performance as well as referee decision making. The 'in-the-action' facility of Dartfish (Dartfish, Fribourg, Switzerland) provides a delayed video feed on the computer screen. Video frames are recorded but are not played back on the computer screen until a pre-defined time afterwards. For example, in an educational setting a pupil can perform a skill and then view their performance of the skill 30s later when it is played on computer screen. This saves time as the system does not require too much user operation once it is set up to provide a delayed feed. The pupil, under the supervision of a teacher, can repeatedly perform the skill, receiving feedback

quantitative and qualitative analysis

from the delayed feed, identifying different things to focus on during subsequent attempts. The teacher may also view the athlete performing the skill live, identifying specific points that need to be considered by the pupil. The teacher can then point these out to the pupil while they both observe the delayed playback of the action on the computer screen.

Video provides a permanent record of performance which can be analysed in detail after performances. Split screen views can be used to view a performance from different angles once videos have been synchronised. Alternatively, the split screen view can be used to display two different performances for the purpose of comparison. These could be two performances by the same athlete or performances of two different athletes.

The Simulcam™ facility of Dartfish allows different performances at the same venue to be shown with one superimposed on the other. This allows a more direct comparison than a split screen view showing the two performances. The image processing software produces a single image for each frame where a blended view is produced by compensating for different camera angles used in the two original video sequences.

Figure 2.1 is a representation of the Stromotion™ facility of Dartfish. Stromotion analyses a video sequence of a player and then produces a single image containing a series of static images of an athlete, or object, displayed on a background constructed from background images within

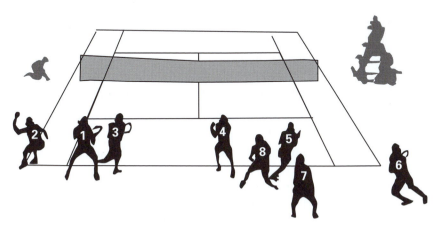

Figure 2.1 Dartfish's Stromotion™ facility

the individual frames of the original video sequence. This type of image can be used to analyse technique during movement or tactical aspects of movement. As well as providing a still image showing an athlete in successive locations, Stromotion can show a video with clip with 'ghost images' of previous locations being shown as the athlete moves to successive locations. The frame locations of these 'ghost images' are adjusted to account for camera zooming and panning.

As has been mentioned in Chapter 1, biomechanical analysis of important sports techniques falls under the broad umbrella of sports performance analysis. Qualitative biomechanics has been used within the study of sports performance (Knudson and Morrison, 2002). Qualitative analysis in biomechanics describes and analyses movements non-numerically by seeing movements as 'patterns' while quantitative analysis describes and analyses movements using numerical measures.

## Strengths

The strength of qualitative analysis of sports performance is that it is done by experienced and expert observers with great knowledge of the sport. They have a 'trained eye' and know what to look for. The expert observer is able to analyse the auditory-visual information they have in a much more unrestricted way than would be the case in objective approaches. Indeed, the analysis can be based on background knowledge and information as well as the information that is directly observed from the performance. Qualitative analysis is based on complex visual and audio information that is more complete than the more abstract representations of performance used in quantitative approaches. The human mind has powerful perceptual ability and capacity for processing very complex information. Detailed information about the quality of technical performance, the context of that performance and the degree of difficulty is lost through the sole reliance on numerical counts, ratings and timings.

Qualitative analysis can be done inexpensively without requiring expensive cameras, computers and sports analysis software. Coaches can observe action in a three dimensional space using perspective and adjusting head position and eye focus as necessary. This may seem like a trivial point. However, the author of this book uses a system to analyse netball live where he has the choice of observing the action on a two dimensional computer screen or naturally looking over the top of the computer screen.

## 36

The author chooses the latter way to observe because it is much easier to distinguish between players and identify the events that need to be recorded.

## Limitations

The limitations of qualitative analysis of performance are related to subjective processes that are involved. These have been used as a rationale for performance analysis support for the coach (Franks and Miller, 1986; Laird and Waters, 2008). The limitations of live qualitative analysis without match recordings include limited recall, observer fatigue, personal bias, emotion and subjective interpretation. Studies of coach recall of critical events during soccer matches have revealed that the accuracy of coach recall is limited. Franks and Miller (1986) found that 42 per cent of critical events could be recalled accurately. A later study by Laird and Waters (2008) found that 59 per cent of critical events were recalled accurately.

We have seen in this section that qualitative methods are not restricted to coach recall without the support of technology and analysts. Video recordings of performances can be used by coaches within a more complete analysis of performance. In such situations, there are still limitations to qualitative analysis that need to be recognised. Observer fatigue can reduce the quality of data recording. The assessment of performance may vary from expert to expert. Qualitative approaches involve personal interpretation of incidents. In soccer, experts, players, managers looking at the same footage of an incident in the penalty area will disagree whether a penalty should have been awarded or not. This seems to happen on a weekly basis and readers are encouraged to think about this as they watch half-time or post-match analysis during sports coverage on television. In many sports, referees have to use interpretation of incidents with respect to the rules of games (Coleclough, 2013). We can expect even more inconsistent interpretation from coaches, players and spectators who have not been trained as referees. More complex issues relating to wider performance and speculation on the tactics chosen by athletes and teams leads to even greater scope for individual interpretation and conclusions drawn by observers.

## AUTOMATICALLY GATHERED DATA

### Object tracking

Hawkeye coaching systems integrate ball tracking technology with biomechanical analysis and video analysis. The system has been used to visually track the trajectory of the ball in tennis and cricket for officiating and broadcast purposes. The system works by using images from multiple cameras within triangulation algorithms. At each point in time, the corresponding two dimensional frames from different cameras are used to form a virtual three dimensional space calculating the ball's location within this. A sequence of frames is used allowing the flight of the ball to be calculated. In tennis, one of the uses of Hawkeye is to determine where the ball struck the playing surface and whether a shot was in or out. As we can see in Figure 2.2, the ball contacting the ground might not be included within the frames recorded by the cameras. Hawkeye operates at 500Hz which means a ball travelling at 263km/h will have an images recorded every 14.6cm. This will be explained in the next paragraph. Despite the discrete and incomplete data recorded, the location at which the ball contacts the ground can be calculated using the predictive models of ball flight given the frames that have been recorded. Some of these frames will be recorded while the ball is travelling towards the playing surface and some will be recorded when the ball is travelling away from the playing surface. A graphic animation is produced of the ball bouncing showing viewers (players, judges, coaches and spectators and television audiences) whether the ball was in or out. The algorithms used are based on assumptions about ball flight and how much of the ball area is in contact with the court when it bounces at different angles and speeds. Hawkeye's website has reported the average error to be 3.6mm (www.hawkeyeinnovations.co.uk/page/sports-officiating/tennis accessed 29 July 2013).

At the time of writing, the fastest recorded serve in professional tennis was 263km/h by Samuel Groth in May 2012 (http://en.wikipedia.org/wiki/Fastest_recorded_tennis_serves, accessed 29 July 2013). This is about $73.1m.s^{-1}$. As shown in Figure 2.3, the length of a tennis court is 23.78m with the shortest serve distance (down the middle) being 18.29m. The frame rate of 500Hz means that there is a frame recorded by each camera every 0.002s. A ball travelling at $73.1m.s^{-1}$ will travel 14.6cm in 0.002s ($0.002s \times 73.1m.s^{-1} = 0.146m$). Remember that the ball does not

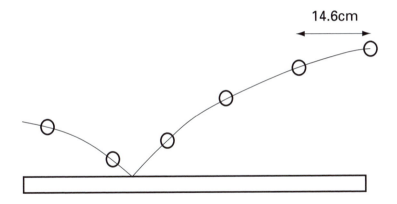

14.6cm

**Figure 2.2** Hawkeye tennis ball tracking

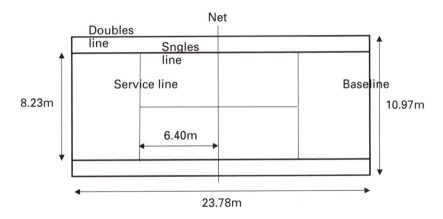

Net

Doubles
line

Sngles
line

Service line

Baseline

8.23m

10.97m

6.40m

23.78m

**Figure 2.3** Dimensions of a tennis court

travel at uniform speed between the impact of the serve and landing on the playing surface. Therefore, the distance of 14.6cm is a mean distance between ball locations in successive frames rather than a universal value when a serve is played at 263km/h.

## Goal line technology

Goal line technology was introduced in English FA Premier League soccer in the 2013–14 season. In the years leading up to its introduction, goal line technology had been a topical issue. FIFA (Fédération Internationale de Football Association) secretary general Jerome Valcke has been reported as stating that systems guaranteeing a 100 per cent success rate would be considered (goal.com 2011, www.goal.com/en-us/news/1786/fifa/2011/03/14/2394555/fifa-open-to-hawk-eye-goal-line-technology accessed 30 July 2013). How feasible is this? The hardest shot recorded in soccer has been reported as being between 84 and 96 miles per hour using different methods (Guardian, 2007 www.theguardian.com/football/2007/feb/14/theknowledge.sport, accessed 29 July 2013). Let's consider a ball crossing the line at 80 miles per hour ($35.8 \text{m.s}^{-1}$) and the whole of the ball is over the whole of the line by 5cm before bouncing back off the goalkeeper who is located behind goal. We will assume the ball rebounds back out of the goal at 40 miles per hour, thus taking twice as long to travel the 5cm as it did on the way into the goal. The whole of the ball is over the whole of the line for 0.001398s prior to the keeper touching the ball ($0.05 \text{m}/35.8 \text{m.s}^{-1}$ = 0.001398s). The ball remains over the whole of the line for a further 0.002796s as it rebounds off the keeper. Therefore, the whole of the ball is over the whole of the line for 0.004195s. With a frame rate of 500Hz, we should see ball every 0.002s so two or three frames should contain images of the whole of the ball being located over the whole of the line. However, the criterion of 100 per cent accuracy means that all possible cases of the whole of the ball being over the whole of the line need to be identified by the technology. What if the ball rebounded off the keeper when it was 1cm over line, or 1mm over the line! In these situations, the expected number of frames where the whole of the ball is located over the whole of the line is 0.420 and 0.042 respectively. Predictive algorithms based on images of the ball travelling towards and away from the goal can be used to estimate whether or not the whole of the ball crossed the whole of the line. These algorithms are based on assumptions in the same way that the algorithms used to determine where a tennis ball bounces rely on assumptions.

## Player tracking

Global positioning technology (GPS) systems can be used to track performers providing a variety of statistical and graphical outputs. The Catapult system (Catapultsports, Melbourne, Victoria, Australia) integrates the GPS data with heart rate data and accelerometer data within a reasonably unobtrusive device that can be worn by players, located near the subscapular. This device is durable and has been used within contact sports. The data can be transferred wirelessly to laptop computers, iPads or iPhones on the side-line of the playing area in real time. The Optimeye S5 device operates at 10Hz and the data can be integrated with ball tracking data. There are other potential player tracking technologies based on directional radio signals and image processing (Carling *et al.*, 2008; Carling and Bloomfield, 2013). Image processing based systems such as Prozone (Prozone Sports Ltd, Leeds, UK) and Amisco (Amisco, Nice, France) are not covered in the current subsection because there is a manual verification process required by quality control personnel (Di Salvo *et al.*, 2009).

## Instrumentation

Any process where data are automatically gathered by equipment without human observer judgement as part of the process is objective. For example, the stroke rates and speeds recorded by the Concept2 rowing ergometer (http://concept2.co.uk/birc/ accessed 30 July 2013) or the electronic recording of split times for marathon runners based on chips within timing tags (London Marathon 2013, www.virginmoneylondon-marathon.com/marathon-centre/virgin-london-marathon-information/your-timing-tag/ accessed 30 July 2013) are totally objective. Note that being totally objective does not mean that the data are necessarily totally accurate; it simply means that there is no subjective judgement as part of the process. There are other sports measuring apparatus used to measure distances in field athletics that would not count as totally objective, because a judge is needed to place a marker at the point where an object is perceived to have landed. Similarly, the computerised scoring system used in amateur boxing (until 2014) requires human operation which clearly involves subjective judgement and would not count as totally objective.

## Quantitative biomechanics

Biomechanics is a discipline of sports science in its own right with methodologies and theory that integrate anatomy, mechanical principles and motor control. Some biomechanics work fits within the scope of sports performance analysis where actual sports performance is being studied. Due to the practical problems of using invasive methods during actual competition, much quantitative biomechanics work is done in laboratory settings. Where important skills of the sport such as the serve in tennis or golf swing are being analysed, the data gathered are considered to be about performance of the actual sports skills (O'Donoghue, 2010: 2). Quantitative biomechanics uses automatic data gathering systems that track markers on athletes being tested. These systems include Vicon (Vicon motion systems, Oxford, UK) where multiple sensors track reflective markers placed on athletes' bodies.

## Strengths

The main advantage of totally automated systems is that there is no subjective human classification of movement or behaviour during the process of data gathering. This does not necessarily mean that systems are accurate, but it does mean that they are free of perceptual errors that can be made by human operators. Biomechanical analysis systems, such as Vicon, allow very detailed information to be gathered allowing finer assessments to be made than when expert human observation of technique is done. Smoothing algorithms can be applied to remove noise in the raw recorded data.

Automated object and player tracking systems offer accurate recording of larger volumes of information than would be the case with human operators. This makes studies more efficient and representative of the sport through using more players.

## Limitations

There are limitations in using automatic biomechanical analysis systems. They are very costly and typically require participants to travel to special purpose biomechanics laboratories. It is not practical to set up equipment

42

at competition venues and the use of reflective markers is invasive. Marker placement is important and can impact on the validity of information produced by systems. The results can be difficult to understand for many practitioners, although innovations in visualisation have seen great improvements in this area in recent years. Quantitative analysis of measured parameters can be 'overkill' and miss important environmental information and other relevant factors (Knudson, 2013: 6).

Object tracking systems such as Hawkeye need to be set up carefully as any slight misplacement of a camera can lead to inaccurate recording of ball location. Player tracking systems can suffer from similar problems if they assume playing surfaces are completely flat. Soccer pitches often rise towards the centre circle to assist drainage.

Where an automatic player tracking system records player location accurately and frequently (for example at 10Hz), it is possible to estimate distance covered, speed and acceleration of movement. Consider Figure 2.4 which shows an example of player movement (the dashed line) and the locations of the player recorded every 0.1s during this movement. The actual path between successive locations for the player is unknown to the player tracking system which assumes the player travels in straight lines between points. Even if some curve fitting algorithm is used, the system cannot be sure of the actual path of movement taken by the player.

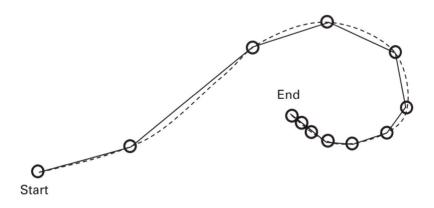

**Figure 2.4** Player movement on playing surface (the dashed line represents actual movement while the solid represents estimated movement)

Considering Figure 2.4, we can see that the accuracy can be improved if locations are recorded more frequently (e.g. 20Hz). If the system records locations less frequently (there are some player tracking systems that operate at 1Hz) then the locations and distance information will be less accurate. The inaccuracies in distances covered will translate into further inaccuracies as velocities and accelerations are estimated.

Many player tracking systems record player location without recording the aspect (direction) faced by a player. A player moving a 4m.s$^{-1}$ might be jogging forward, rapidly shuffling backwards or skipping sideways. The intensity of movement depends on the direction the player is moving in as well as the speed of movement. Moving backwards or sideways would be expected to extract a higher energy cost than moving forward at the same speed. Where playing tracking systems do not distinguish between forward, backward and sideways movement, analysis of data may underestimate the percentage of time that players spend perform- ing high intensity activity. For example, the percentage of time soccer players spend moving at 4m.s$^{-1}$ or faster is about 7 per cent (Redwood- Brown *et al.*, 2012). The speed of 4m.s$^{-1}$ is quite slow by athletic standards; equivalent to 25s for 100m, 1 minute 40s for a lap of a 400m track, 6 minutes 42s per mile. Subjective analysis of work-rate in soccer has suggested that players spend 10 per cent of the match performing high intensity activity (O'Donoghue *et al.*, 2005b). It is most likely that there is some movement performed at 4m.s$^{-1}$ or faster that would not be classified as high intensity activity by expert observers. However, some activity performed at speeds of less than 4m.s$^{-1}$ is classified as high inten- sity activity by expert observers. This activity includes high intensity shuffling movements performed on the spot or in backwards or sideways directions as well as vertical movement to compete for aerial balls. The amount of high intensity activity performed at speeds less than 4m.s$^{-1}$ may be greater than the amount of low intensity activity performed at speeds of 4m.s$^{-1}$ or faster. This explains the difference between the values for percentage of time spent performing high intensity activity of 10 per cent derived from subjective classification and 7 per cent based on a threshold speed of 4m.s$^{-1}$ for automatic player tracking.

Threshold speeds are used to provide estimates for different locomotive activities. For example, we may use a threshold speed of 2m.s$^{-1}$ to distin- guish walking from jogging, a threshold speed of 4.5m.s$^{-1}$ to distinguish jogging from cruising and a threshold speed of 7m.s$^{-1}$ to distinguish cruis- ing from running. For example, Gregson *et al.* (2010) used 5.5m.s$^{-1}$ as the

44

lower threshold for high speed running and 7m.s$^{-1}$ as the lower threshold for sprinting. Some players may be fitter than others and can jog at speeds that would require other players to run. Systems such as Prozone address this by permitting users to establish player specific thresholds for locomotive movements. However, Siegle and Lames (2010) have shown that the range of speeds that an individual player uses for different locomotive movements overlap. This is illustrated in Figure 2.5. Siegle and Lames (2010) classified movement accordingly as follows:

- Walking: One foot has contact to the ground; there is no flight phase with two feet off.
- Jogging: Moving at a slow monotonous pace.
- Cruising: Manifest purpose and effort, usually when gaining distance.
- Sprinting: Maximal effort, rapid motion.

These movements were recorded by human observers. Siegle and Lames (2010) then accessed the movement speeds of players according to a player tracking system at times where they had been recorded as performing different locomotive movements. There was a range of speeds used for each locomotive movement which were analysed and presented as normal distributions of speeds based on the mean and standard deviation of the observed speeds. This suggested an overlap in the speed ranges used to perform different locomotive movements as shown in Figure 2.5. The overlap in movement speeds used for walking and jogging can be explained by the range of purposes of each activity. Walking during a soccer match can range from slow single stepping while maintaining a location when the ball is in the other half of the field to brisker walking where the player knows the location they need to be in to take a throw in, for example. Similarly jogging can be performed at speeds less than 2m.s$^{-1}$ when a player breaks into a jog but wishes to move slow enough to avoid committing to moving to a specific location or in a specific direction. Jogging can also be performed at speeds greater than 4m.s$^{-1}$ where players are moving with an intention of reaching a specific location but without exerting themselves to the extent that they would be cruising or sprinting. The ability to change direction is related to movement speed (Grehaigne et al., 1997) as players have greater scope to change direction when moving at lower speeds. There is a tradeoff between how far a player can move from their current location and how much they can change direction that are both influenced by the current movement speed. The faster a player is moving, the further they can go

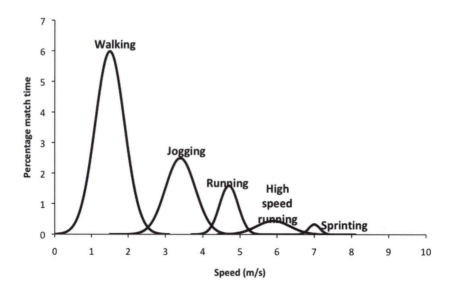

Figure 2.5 Range of speeds at which different locomotive movements are performed

in the next one second, but the slower a player is moving, the greater the scope for changing direction. This leads to locomotive movements being performed at a range of speeds. Players may deliberately jog or cruise with shortened stride length to help change direction if they need to react to opponent play. Moving with the ball (dribbling) requires the player to periodically touch the ball with one or other foot which results in variance from normal locomotive movement which may also influence the speed of movement.

## QUANTITATIVE ANALYSIS OF QUALITATIVE DATA

### Traditional notational analysis

Notational analysis, whether manual or computerised, has traditionally involved subjective judgement at the point of data collection. Consider the time-motion analysis example that was introduced in Chapter 1. We will consider the seven movement classification version here. We end up with a numerical frequency for the number of jogs and the number

quantitative and qualitative analysis

of runs performed by a player. We also end up with a numerical value for the mean duration of jogging instances and the mean duration of running instances. However, at the point of data collection when we are entering the start of instances into the computerised system, there was a subjective decision being made as to whether the player under observation was jogging, running or performing some other movement. This is illustrated in Figure 2.6 where there are two observers; one verbally coding the movement of a player and the other pressing function keys corresponding to the verbally coded activity.

The process involves individual perception of movement. The sporting background of the observer may influence what they consider to be jogging and running. An observer with a background in athletics may limit running to movement being performed at higher speeds than would be applied by observers from game playing backgrounds. A background in athletics means that the observer is used to watching athletes running with full mental and physical effort focused on forward motion. Where a games player runs while looking for space, watching where opponents are, where team-mates are and where the ball is, the observer from an athletics background might be a bit more reluctant to refer to it as running than others would be.

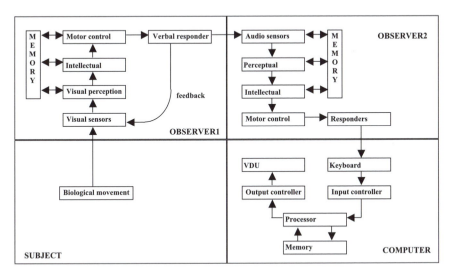

Figure 2.6 Model human information processor

Another example is the computerised scoring system used (until recently) in amateur boxing where judges press a red (blue) button where they perceive the boxer in red (blue) to have thrown a scoring punch. Where three or more of the five judges press a button of the same colour within one second, a point is awarded to the boxer concerned. The fact that there are occasions where one, two, three, or four of the five judges press the same button is evidence that the judging method involves subjective processes, reaction time differences and data entry errors (Coalter *et al.*, 1998). A scoring punch is one made with the white knuckle part of the glove, striking the front of the head or torso with the weight of the shoulder behind the punch. This is not a precise definition that can be executed identically by different judges watching the same bout. The system comes up with a score based on button pressing activity of the judges. However, the numerical score is derived from activity where subjective processes have been involved.

There is an additional issue with the counting of scoring punches that would be an issue even if the five judges were in 100 per cent agreement about the scoring punches made by each boxer. The number of scoring punches made by a boxer is just a quantitative count without any detail of the quality of the punch. The computerised scoring system has a disadvantage in this respect when comparing it to an alternative where experienced judges use their knowledge and expertise to decide on the winner. The computerised scoring system itself changed the nature of amateur boxing and the boxers maximise their chance of winning according to this scoring system. For example, the use of combinations may be counter-productive if the system can only record one scoring punch in a period of one second. If a boxer lands three punches that satisfy the criteria for being a scoring punch within one second, but the opponent is able to land one scoring punch in response during this period, it is possible that each boxer will score a single point. A strategy based on making single scoring punches at a time while avoiding conceding a scoring punch would seem more effective.

There are ways to improve the objectivity of traditional notation systems through providing guidance to observers. For example, we can give descriptions for movement to be classified as walking, jogging, cruising and sprinting as Siegle and Lames (2010) did. Another example is the definition of net points in tennis which could be defined as points where a player crosses the service line when there are still one or more shots to be played in the rally.

48

## Unenforceable definitions

There are some definitions which are quite specific but which cannot be implemented with precision by a human observer. For example, we might specify a speed threshold of 4m.s⁻¹ to distinguish jogging from running. Any forward movement faster than walking but slower than 4m.s⁻¹ is counted as jogging. Any forward movement performed at 4m.s⁻¹ or faster is counted as running. In this example, running and sprinting are merged into a single running category. It is very difficult for a human observer to recognise the point in time when an accelerating or decelerating player reaches 4m.s⁻¹. The definition may exist, but observers cannot apply it accurately. A further issue here is that the choice of 4m.s⁻¹ as a threshold value distinguishing jogging and running is arbitrary. Why not 3.87ms⁻¹? Why not 4.04ms⁻¹? Should we be using the same threshold value for all surface conditions? Should we be using the same value in the second half as is used in the first half? Should we be recognising lower speeds than 4m.s⁻¹ when the player is accelerating from rest?

Another example of operational definitions that cannot be precisely implemented by human observers is direction of passes made in an invasive team game. We could use 90° sectors to represent forward, backward, left and right directions of passes as shown in Figure 2.7. This is unambiguous but where a pass is played diagonally, it will be difficult to determine which of two sectors the pass was in. A further consideration

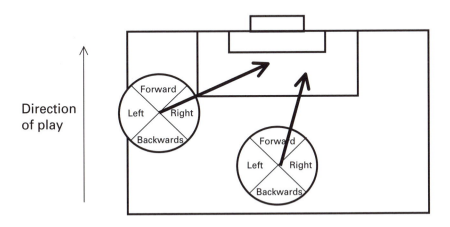

**Figure 2.7** Pass directions

is that definition itself might not be appropriate especially where a player is in on the left or right wing of the playing area and playing a diagonal ball into the attacking area. According to the definition used, some passes like this may be diagonal but in terms of the tactics of the game they cannot be counted the same as passes played in the same direction from other areas of the playing surface.

## Strengths

The quantitative analysis of subjectively classified events manages the complexity of sports performance providing an abstract representation of the performance that aids decision making. Traditional notation methods combine quantitative techniques while also benefiting from expert observer judgement. The systems used are also less costly than automatic player tracking systems.

## Limitations

There are times where precise definitions result in measuring something other than what we intended. Imagine that we are recording rally lengths in tennis to evaluate work-rate. To be objective, we could define the rally as starting when the server strikes the ball (assuming the serve is going to land in and is not a clean ace). We could also define the end point of a rally as when the point ends according to the rules of tennis. The rally may end where an error is played; the ball strikes the net or lands somewhere other than the opponent's half of the court. The other way that the rally may end is when a winner is played. The point has not ended until the ball bounces twice without the opponent reaching it with the racket. Imagine a point where one player serves and the opponent reaches it but as the return is played, the ball goes high in the air and is obviously not going to land in. The rally has effectively ended at this point and both players will be able to relax and prepare for the next point. However, the rally is not recorded as having ended until the return of serve does indeed land out. Similarly, a player may play a smash at the net and as soon as the ball bounces for the first time, it is clear that the opponent will not be able to reach it before it bounces for a second time. In this sense, being objective may over-estimate the amount of work that players do in tennis. Skilled observers will be able to reliably record rally lengths according

50

to the definition given. However, this is the official rally length rather than a period of intense work which might have ceased sooner.

The classification of behaviour, while managing complexity in sports performance, does come with the disadvantage of different behaviours being included in the same broad behaviour class. Consider the seven movement classification scheme used in time-motion analysis (stationary, walking, backing, jogging, running including sprinting, shuffling and game-related activity). In particular, consider the use of game-related activity which is defined as any movement with the ball or challenging for the ball during live game time. Imagine you are using the system on a computer with a different function key used to represent each movement. You are watching a forward. The ball comes towards the forward and you are already anticipating that you will have to enter game-related activity. As he receives the ball, you press the function key to record that the player has started to engage in game-related activity. He dribbles the ball towards goal, under pressure from opposing defenders, who he evades until, nine seconds after receiving the ball, he has a shooting opportunity and shoots for goal. As he shoots, he skips to the side and you enter the function key for shuffling and continue to record his activity for the rest of the match period. So a nine-second instance of game-related activity has been entered. Now imagine you are using the same system at another match when observing a defender. An opposition attack has just been unsuccessful and the keeper has the ball. Players on both teams start to walk or jog up the field. The defender walks, turns around to face the goalkeeper and steps backwards away from his goal making himself available to receive the ball. No opposing players are near the defender as he is deep in his own half and no immediate threat to their goal. The goalkeeper rolls the ball towards the defender. The defender receives the ball and you press the function key to record that the defender has started to engage in game-related activity according to our definition. The defender walks forward, controlling the ball in front of him, looking up field looking for the best option to play the ball up field. The opposing players give him space and do not come forwards to pressurise him. The defender keeps moving forward with another touch of the ball and another touch and then, nine seconds after initially receiving the ball from the goalkeeper, he plays the ball into the opposing half of the field. You press the function key to indicate that the defender is now jogging forwards having played the ball up field. According to our system, the attacking player in the first match and the defender in the second match have spent nine seconds performing the same activity. The intensity of the forward's nine-second instance of game-related activity would have been higher than that of the defender's. This is a limitation of the system which tries to use a small number of movement classes to represent the full complexity of playing soccer.

Let us consider another example in time-motion analysis which comes from some players being fitter than others. Imagine that you are using the seven movement classification system to record the activity of a midfielder. His team has just mounted an attack and the ball has gone out of play for a goal kick to the opposing team. The outfield players of both teams make their way to the central third of the field. You have pressed the function key for running because the midfielder appears to be finding moving at his current speed taxing and is breathing heavily. You continue to watch, waiting for the midfielder to slow down to a jog as he reaches the location where he wants to be when the goal kick is taken. As he is still running, you notice an opposing player jogging along-side him at the same speed even though the midfielder is running. The issue here is that both players (the midfielder and the opponent) are moving at the same speed. It is a jog for one of them, but requires the other to make an effort that is greater than if jogging. We may be analysing the player as part of a study of many players to understand the demands of the game. We have recorded that the midfielder is running, but that is only because this speed of movement required him to break into a run rather than jogging as some other players are able to. The player may not be as fit as others and it is undeniable that soccer players have a range of fitness levels. So when analysing this player, we may end up with a higher figure for the percentage of time spent performing high intensity activity than for other players simply because the game requires him to work harder than others. In this situation, it is best to analyse what is required for the player under observation and hopefully, if we include enough players in the study, the activity of the fitter players will be balanced against that of the less fit players. Trying to make judgements about what is required for the 'average player' when observing a fit (or less fit) player will simply add to the difficulty of the analysis task.

A third example is taking a shot in football. Imagine you are using the two movement classification scheme (work and rest) while observing a forward. You use one function key on the computer when you perceive the player to commence high intensity activity and another when you perceive the player to be performing low to moderate intensity activity.

It does not matter whether the ball is in play or whether it is stoppage time. It does not matter whether the player has the ball or not at any instance. All that matters is whether the player is perceived to be working at a high intensity or not. The player is walking, then slowly jogging, clearly not requiring high intensity effort. He is about 30m away from the opposition goal when the ball comes across field towards him from the wing. He takes a shot but in so doing he seems to casually swing his leg at the ball and, in a moment of hesitation, you fail to press the work function key and the player continues to jog slowly after taking the shot. You consider what has just happened and wonder whether the shot required high intensity effort. It seemed to be so easy for the player and yet the ball moved very quickly towards goal once struck. You know that you, yourself, would have to strike the ball very vigorously, undoubtedly with high intensity effort to make it move that fast. Even though the forward under observation made it look easy, striking the ball with one of his bandy muscular legs, it would have required mechanical work. This is another example of whether we are analysing the demands of the game independently of particular players' fitness levels or whether we are analysing the effort required for the particular players we observe. A study of high intensity activity in soccer would need to include a sufficient number of players so that the average results would be representative of the demands of the game.

## EVENTS WHERE DECISIONS ARE INDEPENDENT OF THE ANALYST

There are objective observational methods where the observers are not required to make subjective judgements. In such methods, other individuals such as umpires or referees or event technological aids make decisions. For example, in tennis, an observer may simply enter the outcome of a point according to the match officials. If a ball is called out, the observer enters this irrespective of whether the observer viewed the ball as landing in or out. Where the challenge system in tennis is used, the outcome determined by the system is recorded by the observer rather than the outcome the observer felt should have happened. There may be perceptual errors made by match officials; for example the incidents where goals are given in soccer where the whole of the ball did not cross the whole of the line as well as incidents where a goal is not given when the whole of the ball has crossed the whole of the line. There is, however, no additional error made by the analyst who is accurately recording the decisions made by others. Such systems need to use decisions made by persons with expertise responsible for important roles such as umpires and referees. Data recorded by other analysts or journalists would not count as such a method.

While some studies have been done using purely service calls and point outcomes according to umpires (O'Donoghue, 2013b), it is more typical in sports performance analysis for a mixture of variable types to be used. Some will involve operator judgement while others will not. There are some events in sports performance that are more 'matter of fact' than others. Table 2.2 shows variables with differing levels of objectivity in tennis. The different degrees of objectivity of such variables can be expressed using reliability statistics as we will see in Chapter 9.

**Strengths**

The main strength of using data where decisions are made by umpires or referees rather than analysts is the expertise and ability of those making the decisions. The quality of the data will be good due to the

Table 2.2 Objectivity of variables recorded during tennis points

| Objective | Variable | Explanation |
| --- | --- | --- |
| Yes | Ace | Umpire's decision |
| Yes | Double fault | Umpire's decision |
| Yes | Point winner | Umpire's decision |
| Yes | Service (1st or 2nd) | Umpire's decision |
| Usually Yes | Point ending (winner or error) | Some coaches count some forced errors as winners |
| Expected Yes | Ground stroke type (forehand or backhand) | Reasonably obvious |
| Expected No | Third of the service box where serve landed | Judgement of location |
| No | Point type (baseline or net) | Interpretation of guidelines |
| No | Serve type (flat, slice or kick) | Requires expert observers |
| No | Error type (forced or unforced) | Observer judgement |

important role of officiating sports contests. Game state may be of interest for coaches or analysts studying performance in different scorelines. Where the opinions of analysts and umpires differ, using umpires' decisions ensures the score recorded is the same as that experienced by the players.

## Limitations

There are limitations to using the decisions of umpires when recording events performed in sports contests. The first disadvantage is that relying exclusively on such variables excludes important variables about tactics and skills performed. The second disadvantage is that in some sports, referees need to interpret rules when making decisions and this can be done inconsistently within some sports (Coleclough, 2013). Indeed there are performance analysis bureaus that monitor the decisions made by referees. The referees have to make decisions during the game, often without the assistance of technology. The bureaus reviewing referee performance use post-match video analysis where repeated viewing of incidents is done to maximise the accuracy of feedback being given to referees.

## SUMMARY

Sports performance can be analysed using qualitative methods as well as quantitative methods. Qualitative analysis can be subjective but also uses coaching expertise and knowledge. Quantitative methods avoid human judgements as far as possible. Some systems are totally objective with no human involvement in data collection. Traditional notational analysis does involve human observation which requires guidelines and a need to certify the level of reliability of the data. Both quantitative and qualitative methods have their strengths and weaknesses.

# CHAPTER 3

## SPORTS PERFORMANCE DATA AND INFORMATION

### INTRODUCTION

Chapter 2 covered quantitative and qualitative data and introduced some of the analysis methods used with these types of data. The purpose of this chapter is to describe the different types of data and information involved in sports performance analysis. Central to the chapter is the discussion of performance indicators and their use in sports performance analysis. The chapter will describe what performance indicators are, their properties and their relationship with the other types of data and information used in sports performance analysis. A number of different ways of interpreting performance indicator values are also described in the chapter. This chapter covers the raw data that are captured during sports performance analysis and how performance indicators are derived from those data. The detail of system processes that perform this transformation of data will be covered in Chapters 4 to 8. The key measurement issue being addressed by this chapter is validity. Any analysis system should produce information that is relevant allowing coaches and players to make informed decisions about important areas of performance. The chapter describes how students can use coaching literature in sports of interest to determine the most relevant information to use.

### THE REDUCTIVE APPROACH

Sports performance is highly complex and capable of generating vast quantities of data. This is the case for all sports, especially team games.

56

One of the main tasks of sports performance analysis is to reduce the full complexity of sports performance to a manageable volume of information that can be used to support decisions. This involves abstraction; forming a representation of sports performance that contains the most important information and excludes unnecessary noise. Figure 3.1 gives an idea of the reductive approach used within sports performance analysis. Let us consider the example of a tennis match. The first stage of reducing the information is video recording the match. The video recording contains a vast amount of information in each video frame. Despite this, the video recording still excludes a great deal of relevant performance information experienced by the performers, atmospheric information experienced by those present and many potential views of the performance not covered by the video cameras present. Data can be recorded for each point played in the match, for example:

- The score in sets, games and points at the beginning of the point
- Who served
- Whether the first serve was in or not
- The placement of the serve (left, middle or right of the target service court)
- The number of shots played
- The type of point (ace, serve winner, double fault, return winner, net point or baseline rally)
- How the point ended (winner, forced error or unforced error)
- The player who won the point

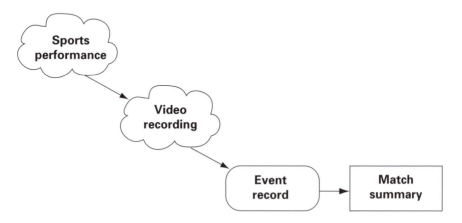

Figure 3.1 Data reduction in sports performance analysis

This is an abstract representation of a point using a fingerprint of eight data items. There is a great deal of information that is excluded from this abstract representation. Information about individual shots could have been recorded; where they were played from, whether forehand or backhand, whether volley or groundstroke, where the ball landed, pace of the shot, information about shot mechanics, spin, etc., could all have been recorded. The abstract representation of the tennis point also excludes information about player movement between shots and while playing shots. There is still a large volume of information recorded because a tennis match is made up of many points. Consider the 2012 US Open men's singles final between Andy Murray and Novak Djokovic; there were 315 points played over this five-set match. Therefore, a further process of data reduction is needed to transform the data for individual points into an overall match summary such as that shown in Table 3.1. This match summary is provided on the tournament's official website along with additional information summarising serve direction and individual shot types played with the forehand and backhand (approach shots, drop shots, ground strokes, lobs, overhead shots, passing shots and volleys).

The information in Table 3.1 is a performance profile because it is a collection of relevant aspects of tennis performance including serving, receiving, break points, winners and errors. The term 'profiling' in sports

Table 3.1 Overall match summary of 2012 US Open men's singles final (www.usopen.org accessed 31 December 2012)

| Match statistic | Andy Murray | Novak Djokovic |
| --- | --- | --- |
| Aces | 5 | 7 |
| Double faults | 4 | 5 |
| 1st serves in | 98 of 150 = 65% | 103 of 165 = 62% |
| 1st serve points won | 61 of 98 = 62% | 65 of 103 = 63% |
| 2nd serve points won | 25 of 52 = 48% | 26 of 62 = 42% |
| Fastest serve | 132 MPH | 128 MPH |
| Average 1st serve speed | 111 MPH | 116 MPH |
| Average 2nd serve speed | 83 MPH | 91 MPH |
| Net points won | 16 of 24 = 67% | 39 of 56 = 70% |
| Break points won | 8 of 17 = 47% | 9 of 18 = 50% |
| Receiving points won | 74 of 170 = 44% | 64 of 154 = 42% |
| Winners | 31 | 40 |
| Unforced errors | 56 | 65 |
| Total points won | 160 | 155 |

58

science is used consistently in this way within other disciplines such as sports psychology and strength and conditioning. In sports psychology, the profile of mood states includes six different components of mood (McNair *et al.*, 1971) and, in strength and conditioning, a fitness profile will contain relevant variables for flexibility, speed, power, endurance and coordination. These profiles are concise manageable abstract portrayals of mood and fitness of an athlete respectively. The sports performance profile shown in Table 3.1 is for an individual performance, but profiles can also be produced for typical performances of players based on multiple match data. Multiple match profiles can also show the spread of performances for an athlete who may be consistent or erratic with respect to some aspects of performance (O'Donoghue, 2005a).

In discussing this reductive approach, we should not lose sight of the fact that the video recording of performance is still very important in sports performance analysis. The match statistics allow aspects of performance requiring attention to be quickly identified. They help identify 'what' the problem areas are and 'what' aspects are being performed well. Armed with this evidence, coaches and players will then view relevant video sequences in detail discussing why the performance is as it is, what could have been done, what alternative decisions may need to be taken and how performance in these areas can improve (O'Donoghue and Mayes, 2013a). The interactive sports video analysis systems available today allow video to be tagged with events which are analysed using the system and summarised as statistics. The systems have the flexibility to allow relevant video sequences to be rapidly identified and replayed. In viewing the video sequences, coaches and players get into the 'why' and the 'how' of performance using a great deal of complex qualitative information that is derived from the video sequences.

In this sense, different types of data are used in different types of analysis. The performance analyst produces and deals with a very restricted set of summary quantitative data. In so doing, the analyst will also use pre-decided targets, performance trend information, performance norms and other knowledge that allow the quantitative information to be interpreted effectively. This basic analysis then focuses the attention of the players and coaches on the important areas. The coaches' and players' analysis of the video sequences uses much more complex information which is supported by their greater knowledge of the sport. Very often analysts might never have competed in the sport they are analysing whereas the sport is a way of life for the players and coaches who have competed and potentially coached and umpired the game at various levels as well. They will have in-depth knowledge of principles of play, tactical options as well as characteristics of good and not so good play. This knowledge is utilised by players and coaches while they analyse relevant video sequences and make decisions about preparation for future matches.

## TERMINOLOGY

### Values and variables

There are many types of data used in sports performance analysis including facts, images, video footage and verbal information. Quantitative data include nominal events, ordinal data and numerical data. In order to understand quantitative data, we need to distinguish between values and variables. Table 3.2 shows some examples from sports performance analysis grouped according to their scale of measurement. A nominal scale is one where there are a finite number of named values such as the different classes of point shown in Table 3.2. These nominal values have no order; they are just different classes of point. An ordinal scale is one where the values have an order such as quality of execution where 'excellent' is a higher quality of execution than 'good' which, in turn, is a higher quality of execution than 'average'. The order of variables allows comparisons such as 'greater than' or 'less than' to be made between values.

Numerical scale variables can have an infinite number of values. Even if values are restricted being between 1 and 2, there are an infinite number of values between 1 and 2 if we use an unrestricted number of decimal places. The scale is continuous between these points. There are two types of numerical scale although some statistical analysis packages merge these as they share many common analysis procedures. The two numerical scales are ratio scale and interval scale. An interval scale is one where there is a fixed interval between unit values. For example the difference between 0 and 1 is 1 as is the difference between 1 and 2 and the difference between 2 and 3. This allows differences between values to be reasoned about through subtraction. Examples of interval scale measures are joint angles in technique analysis. The range of potential values may include negative values with zero being an angle in the middle of the range of angles rather than an absolute zero measure. This makes division of values invalid because we could have division by zero errors.

A ratio scale variable has all of the properties of interval scale variables but also has a zero point that represents an absent of the concept being measured. An example of a ratio scale measure is distance covered in Table 3.2. A value of 0m means that the player has not moved. The zero point representing an absence of the concept of interest allows ratios between values to be reasoned about through division. For example 10,000m is twice the distance that 5,000m is. The variable rating, in Table

Table 3.2 Variables and values of different measurement scales

| Scale of measurement | Variable | Values |
|---|---|---|
| Nominal event | Point class | Ace, Double Fault, Serve Winner, Return Winner, Baseline rally, Net point |
| | Area of field | Defensive 3rd Left Side, Defensive 3rd Middle, Defensive 3rd Right Side, Middle 3rd Left Side, Middle 3rd Middle, Middle 3rd Right Side, Attacking 3rd Left Side, Attacking 3rd Middle, Attacking 3rd Right Side |
| | Netball player | GK, GD, WD, C, WA, GA, GS |
| Ordinal | Quality of execution | Excellent, Good, Average, Poor, Very Poor |
| | Outcome of possession | Goal, shot on target, shot off target, entered attacking third but no opportunity, unsuccessful |
| Interval | Joint angle | −0.5 rad, +0.25 rad |
| Ratio | % Possessions leading to goal | 50.0%, 62.4%, 34.7% |
| | Duration of locomotive movement | 3.5s, 12.4s, 6.2s |
| | Distance covered | 10424m, 11562m |
| | Shots per rally | 17, 2, 1, 6 |
| | Mean shots per rally | 6.2, 5.0, 4.9 |
| | Median shots per rally | 6, 5, 5.5 |
| | Mode shots per rally | 5, 4 |

3.2, is ordinal rather than ratio scale because the numbers are simply numeric codes used to represent ratings rather than points with equal interval in between.

Variables allow us to discuss concepts without having to look at every possible case that is relevant. For example, we can use equation (3.1) for mean rally duration instead of showing the calculation for all values from all possible tennis matches.

Mean rally duration = total time spent in rallies / number
of rallies played                                                                         (3.1)

## DATA AND INFORMATION

The purpose of this section of the chapter is to make clear how the terms data and information are used in sports performance analysis. The terms 'data' and 'information' are not terms that can be used interchangeably as each has a different meaning with respect to any process of data analysis. When we have a process, the input to that process is referred to as 'data' and the output to that process is referred to as 'information'. Figure 3.2 shows a pipeline of four processes that reduce a database of recorded coach behaviour events to a set of summary results. There is an overall

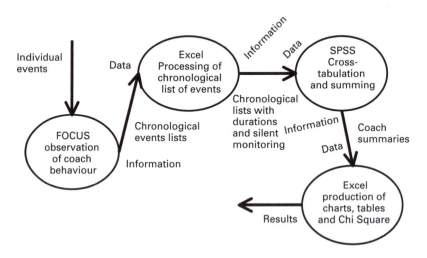

Figure 3.2 Data and information within a pipeline of processes

input (individual events) and an overall output (results) as well as three data flows in between pairs of processes. Each of these three data flows are both data and information. They are information with respect to the processes that output them and data with respect to other processes that use them as inputs. For example, 'coach summaries' is information produced by the third process of the pipeline and data entered into the final process of the pipeline.

The purpose of the processes is to transform data into summary information which they pass directly to other processes or to repositories where data are stored. The repositories could be paper based forms or computer files depending on the system. Similarly, the processes involved in a sports performance analysis system may be manual tasks, automated tasks or a combination of both. An example of a combined task is where a computerised system is used to record data but is operated by a human analyst. Of course, this could be represented by two separate processes (one for human data entry and one for processing the data entered) but such an approach can lead to cumbersome system diagrams.

## Performance indicators and action variables

A performance indicator is a variable used to characterise an aspect of performance that is relevant and important. The properties that distinguish a performance indicator from any other variable about a performance are:

- It must represent some valid and important aspect of the sport.
- It has an objective measurement process.
- There is a known scale of measurement.
- There is a means of interpreting the value of a performance indicator.

Table 3.3 gives examples of tennis performance indicators for different purposes of performance analysis. Technical effectiveness includes measures such as percentage success and winner to error ratios. Let us consider 'first serve performance'. This is not a performance indicator because it is too vague. It is an aspect of performance that still needs to be operationalised. When we operationalise a variable, we define it objectively so that it can be measured consistently by different observers and is independent of observer opinion. Two performance indicators are

Table 3.3 Performance indicators and action variables in tennis

| Purpose of performance analysis | Aspect of | Performance indicator performance | Action variables |
|---|---|---|---|
| Technical effectiveness | First serve performance | % points where first serve was in | Whether the first serve was in |
| | | % points won when first serve was in | Whether the first serve was in |
| | | | Whether the server won the point |
| | Serving effectiveness to advantage court | % points won when serving to advantage court | Court served to |
| | | | Whether the server won the point |
| | Effectiveness at the net | % points won when at the net | Whether the player went to the net |
| | | | Whether the player won the point |
| Tactics | Serve tactics | % points served to left of target service court | The area of the service court where the serve landed |
| | | % points served to middle of target service court | The area of the service court where the serve landed |
| | | % points served to right of target service court | The area of the service court where the serve landed |
| | Net tactics | % points where player went to the net | Whether the player went to the net |
| Physical | Rally length | Mean rally length (s) | Rally length of individual rallies (s) |
| | | % rallies that are longer than 10s | Rally length of individual rallies (s) |

shown for this aspect of performance; the percentage of points where the first serve is in and the percentage of points won when the first serve is in. These two performance indicators are measured on percentage scales and yield values that are understood by coaches and players. Once we have devised such performance indicators, we can identify the raw event data that need to be collected to permit performance indicators to be computed. Going back to the example of the US Open men's singles final where there were 315 points played, we need to know the total number of points each player served, how many of those saw the first serve played in, and how many of those first serve points were won by the server. The need for these totals informs us what facts need to be recorded from each point.

The raw event data that are recorded are referred to as action variables and these can be measured on various scales. For example, who won a point, whether or not a point was a net point, whether or not the first serve was in are all nominal variables. That is they have a restricted set of named values. Whether a point is a net point or not is a straightforward Boolean (true or false) variable as is whether or not the first serve was in and whether or not the serving player won the point.

The length of an individual rally is measured on a ratio scale. A rally length cannot be less than zero and a rally of six seconds is twice as long as a rally of three seconds. Hence a ratio (or division of values) has meaning when we are dealing with variables such as rally length.

Let us consider another example of tactics in soccer where some teams may be reputed to play with a slow build up style of attack while others may be characterised by a more direct style of attacking. Here, the aspect of performance of interest is style of possession play but this is not a performance indicator. It is simply too vague to be a performance indicator. A performance indicator representing this aspect of performance could be the mean number of passes per possession or even the median number of passes per possession.

## Key performance indicators

The term key performance indicator has been used in some literature and in some cases the 'key performance indicators' may be performance indicators but in other cases they are not even performance indicators. Given the qualities of a performance indicator listed in this chapter, key performance indicators need to represent higher order management information that is clearly distinguishable from performance indicators.

## QUALITIES OF PERFORMANCE INDICATORS

### Validity

As has already been mentioned, there are four qualities that a variable must have in order for it to qualify as a performance indicator. The first of these is that it represents some relevant and important aspect of performance; this is validity. There are different ways of determining the validity of a variable; some involving statistical analysis and some are more qualitative. It is not feasible to conduct a statistical analysis of the validity of variables using multiple match data for the purpose of Level 5 coursework. However, there may be some published analyses providing evidence of validity that can be referred to. Similarly, some qualitative techniques might not be feasible either for a Level 5 assignment. I am sure the university soccer coach might not be able interview 20 different students to discuss the main variables of interest in different aspects of soccer.

O'Donoghue (2010: 150–5) discussed different types of validity relevant to sports performance analysis and how these can be evaluated. These are summarised below:

- Logical validity or face validity – this is where the variable is obviously valid, for example the 10,000m finishing time of a 10,000m runner.
- Content validity – is very relevant in performance profiles. A profile has content validity if it consists of performance indicators that cover all relevant aspects of performance.
- Criterion validity – is where a performance indicator for some aspect of performance is evaluated against some gold standard measure for that aspect. The most common type of criterion validity is where performance indicators are correlated with the overall match outcome or performance result.
- Construct validity – applies where some measure is created such as the Eagle rating (Bracewell *et al.*, 2003) and it is necessary to

demonstrate its validity. If the rating variable (for example) clearly distinguishes between performers of known different ability levels then the variable can be considered valid.

■ Decision accuracy – is where the variable can at least distinguish between winners and losers of matches even though the actual recorded value might not be considered a valid measure of performances of different qualities.

Further types of validity that can be added to this list is catalytic validity (Cohen *et al.*, 2011: 187–8) and ecological validity (Cohen *et al.*, 2011: 195). Catalytic validity means that the information produced by a system can be used as an agent for change in practical contexts. In the case of sports performance analysis, this means that the information has a role in performance enhancement. Ecological validity in performance analysis comes from the fact that the information is related to real sports performances.

With respect to criterion validity and construct validity, it is worth noting that a performance indicator may well be valid without being associated with the overall outcome of the performance. The most common types of indicators that may not be associated with performance outcome are tactical indicators. Tactical indicators represent the style of play irrespective of the success with which that style of play is implemented. For example, there may be soccer teams who use slow build up possession styles in all areas of the FIFA World rankings. Similarly, there may be teams who adopt a more direct fast breaking style of possession in all areas of the FIFA World rankings. A performance indicator such as mean number of passes per possession could be used to represent a team's use of possession. There may be considerable overlap between those teams qualifying for the knockout stages of major tournaments and those teams eliminated at the group stages. Indeed, the two distributions of values for this performance indicator may be almost identical between qualifiers and non-qualifiers. This does not mean that it is invalid because the purpose of this indicator is not to distinguish successful and unsuccessful performers but to distinguish teams adopting different strategies. If there are performers reputed to use different tactical styles, then known group difference can still be tested based on reputation for style of play.

As well as statistical comparisons, validity of performance indicators can be evaluated using qualitative techniques. Expert coach opinion of areas of performance can be confirmed prior to operationalising variables to represent these areas. More indirect approaches can also be used; for example, surveying coaching literature to identify important areas of the game to represent by operationalised variables.

## OBJECTIVE MEASUREMENT PROCESS

A variable is objective if its value is independent of a given observer's opinion. Some variables are objective because they do not involve any human activity in their measurement. Such variables include service speeds measured by radar guns, ball tracking variables measured by systems, such as Hawkeye, and movement variables derived from automatic player tracking systems. The objectivity here applies to the action variables being recorded at the individual event level as well as to any match performance indicators ultimately derived from these.

Where human observers are part of the data gathering system, some variables may be made objective by devolving decisions to the match officials. For example, in tennis, we may count a shot as being played in or out based purely on what the umpires and line judges decide in combination with any challenge systems that may be in use. In team games, we may record foul play as having occurred where referees decide that a foul has been committed. This means that the observers will not be exercising any subjective judgement over where shots in tennis landed or whether fouls were committed by players in a team game. While some decisions of match officials may be inaccurate, this does not affect the objectivity of the analysis system being used. Once again, the objectivity here applies at the individual event level and to any performance indicators derived from these events.

There are other variables where human judgement is unavoidable and hence objectivity may be limited. Let us consider the percentage of points where a tennis player makes an unforced error as a performance indicator. This performance indicator will be determined using the nominal point ending data recorded for individual points (winner, forced error or unforced error). The distinction between a winner and an error is obvious where the observer applies the rules of the game of tennis. If the ball lands in court and bounces twice before the opponent can strike it with the racket then the shot is a winner. An error is where a shot lands out of court or is played into the net. There may be some rare points where it is difficult to see whether the opponent reached the ball before it

68

bounced twice, but in these situations the umpire makes the decision as to whether a winner was played or not. The distinction between a forced error and an unforced error is much more difficult to make and requires expert tennis observers. The mental process of deciding if an error was forced or unforced is based on the observer's belief about the chance a player had to play a shot in court. This chance in turn depends on the observer's opinion about the degree of difficulty of the shot based on the location involved, opponent positioning, pace of the ball and spin that might have been applied. In many sports, players use deception and disguise during play. If such deception is capable of deceiving expert players, it will certainly be capable of deceiving non-expert observers. Many experts would argue that the percentage of points where a player makes unforced errors is a valid performance indicator in tennis. Therefore, where expert observers are used, objectivity can be determined by inter-operator agreement studies. There are many other examples of variables requiring subjective judgement in the analysis of tennis. For example, observers may be required to distinguish between flat, slice and kick serve techniques in tennis. In such situations, it is necessary to demonstrate the level of objectivity of the data collection process using inter-operator agreement studies. An issue that remains is the replicability of the data collection process. While the observers used in a particular study or by a particular squad might have demonstrated that they have very good levels of agreement, other readers will not be fully aware of what counted as forced errors, unforced errors, kick serves, slice serves or flat serves without some published guidelines or example video sequences.

There are other occasions where clear definitions are made, but human operators are not capable of applying them when recording events. For example, in tennis we may clearly explain that serves to the left, middle and right of the target service court are based on the service court being divided exactly into three sections. The problem here is that these three sections are not clearly marked on the court and there is no independent match official making decisions at this level of detail. A serve may be played so close to an imaginary line dividing two thirds of a service court that the observer will be unsure which third to record. This is especially true where the serve is played at great speed. In such a situation, it is necessary to demonstrate the strength of inter-operator agreement.

## KNOWN SCALE OF MEASUREMENT

Performance indicators need to have known scales of measurement. This will assist their interpretation. One way of achieving a known scale of measurement is to express event frequencies as a percentage of some total. Let us consider a tennis player who played a three-set first-round match where she served 12 aces and a two-set second-round match where she served nine aces. The raw frequencies are difficult to interpret because tennis matches are of differing lengths. However, if we know that the player played 12 aces out of 100 service points in the first-round match (12.0 per cent) and nine aces out of 60 service points in the second round match (15.0 per cent) then we can see that the percentage of service points that are aces is improving.

Split times in a middle-distance running event are also easier to interpret if we have some known scale of measurement. However, this scale may be relative to the ability of the athlete. Consider an athlete running a 5,000m race who has personal bests of 2 minutes for the 800m, 4 minutes for the 1,500m, 8 minutes 30s for the 3,000m, 15 minutes for the 5,000m and 30 minutes 50s for the 10,000m. These equate to 400m lap times of 60s for the 800m, 64s for the 1,500m, 68s for the 3,000m, 72s for the 5,000m and 74s for the 10,000m. Knowledge of energy systems utilised in different middle-distance and distance athletic events allows us to specify a range of lap times that would be appropriate within a 5,000m race. At World Championship level, 10,000m athletes have produced last laps where they are running at their 800m pace. Therefore, we cannot rule out a lap time of 60s for the athlete under consideration. In a tactical 5,000m race, the athlete could run some laps slower than 10,000m pace. If we assume a slowest lap of 80s, this gives a range of lap times of 20s between 60s and 80s.

### Means of interpretation

The two main ways of interpreting performance indicators are by comparing values to those of opponents within competitions or by comparing values to norms (Hughes and Bartlett, 2002). The idea of comparing values to those of an opponent within the same competition can be extended to comparing performances with one's own values in other situations or periods of the same competition. Table 3.4 shows the serve direction distribution for Andy Murray and Novak Djokovic in the 2012

70

US Open men's singles final. This adds the percentage of points won to the data shown earlier in Table 1.2. This allows us to make some interesting observations that may be useful to the players. For example, Andy Murray had a tendency to serve to more to left (Djokovic's forehand side) on first serve. This was the case when serving to the deuce court and the advantage court. However, the statistics show that Murray was more effective serving to the right hand side in both of these situations (100.0 per cent v. 71.4 per cent to the deuce court and 64.3 per cent v. 50.0 per cent to the advantage court). Tactical variables such as the distribution of serve directions are concerned with decision making. While tactical indicators in isolation reflect tactical decisions irrespective of the effectiveness of play, chosen tactics are often evaluated in terms of the effectiveness of different choices as they have been in Table 3.4.

Table 3.4 allows performances to be considered relative to a player's own performances when serving to other areas of the service court or relative to the performance of the opponent. The alternative approach is to consider a player's performance in relation to norms for the population of performances of interest. This requires the normative data to have been published. Table 3.5 shows decile norms for different performance indicators in tennis. The performance of Novak Djokovic in the final of the men's singles at the 2012 US Open (Table 3.1) can be considered against these norms to see which 10 per cent band of the population of performances each of his values falls into. Table 3.6 shows the raw values as well as the decile bands where Djokovic's performance are located.

There are some of these values where higher values are better, especially the percentage of points won when the first serve is in and the percentage of points won when a second serve is required. There are other variables such as the percentage of service points where double faults are played where lower values are preferable. There are other variables where an optimal value might be preferable. For example, the percentage of points where the first serve is in must not be so low that the player relies on second serve too much and must not be so high that the serve is too easy for an opponent to return. Similarly, a player can play too few net points or too many net points and an optimal value that maximises the percentage of points won at the net might be preferable. One issue that we need to consider with Table 3.6 is that the norms (in Table 3.5) were derived from all Grand Slam competitors but this particular match was played against Andy Murray and performance indicator values might not be as high because of this.

Table 3.4 Serve direction distribution in the US Open men's singles final (points won/points played into court) (www.usopen.org, accessed 31 December 2012)

| Player Service | Deuce | | | Advantage | | |
|---|---|---|---|---|---|---|
| | Left | Middle | Right | Left | Middle | Right |
| Andy Murray | | | | | | |
| 1st | 20/28=71.4% | 4/13=30.8% | 7/7=100.0% | 11/22=50.0% | 10/14=71.4% | 9/14=64.3% |
| 2nd | 0/1=0.0% | 15/28=53.6% | 1/2=50.0% | 0/1=0.0% | 8/14=57.1% | 1/2=50.0% |
| Novak Djokovic | | | | | | |
| 1st | 11/20=55.0% | 8/14=57.1% | 15/21=71.4% | 11/19=57.9% | 5/11=45.5% | 15/18=83.3% |
| 2nd | 4/7=57.1% | 9/19=47.4% | 0/1=0.0% | 1/4=25.0% | 11/24=45.8% | 1/2=50.0% |

Table 3.5 Decile norms for performance indicators in men's singles tennis at the US Open

| Performance indicator | Decile | | | | | | | | |
|---|---|---|---|---|---|---|---|---|---|
| | 10% | 20% | 30% | 40% | 50% | 60% | 70% | 80% | 90% |
| % Points where first serves is in | 52.2 | 54.3 | 56.6 | 58.3 | 60.2 | 62.1 | 63.8 | 66.6 | 69.8 |
| % Points won when 1st serve was in | 57.4 | 62.3 | 64.7 | 66.7 | 69.5 | 71.7 | 74.9 | 77.9 | 83.9 |
| % Points won when a 2nd serve was required | 37.0 | 40.4 | 44.8 | 47.4 | 50.0 | 51.9 | 55.0 | 57.8 | 62.7 |
| % Serving points were aces | 1.2 | 2.6 | 3.5 | 4.9 | 6.3 | 7.1 | 8.7 | 10.5 | 14.4 |
| % Serving points were double faults | 1.1 | 1.4 | 1.9 | 2.4 | 2.9 | 3.5 | 4.1 | 5.1 | 6.2 |
| % Points where player went to net | 4.0 | 5.6 | 6.2 | 7.2 | 7.9 | 9.2 | 10.3 | 11.4 | 13.5 |
| % Net points won | 50.0 | 55.3 | 59.1 | 62.1 | 64.2 | 68.0 | 70.4 | 75.0 | 77.8 |
| Mean first serve speed (km.h$^{-1}$) | 168 | 172 | 174 | 178 | 180 | 182 | 186 | 189 | 193 |
| Mean second serve speed (km.h$^{-1}$) | 132 | 136 | 138 | 140 | 142 | 145 | 149 | 152 | 157 |

Table 3.6 Relating performances to population norms

| Performance indicator | Value | Decile | | | | | | | | |
|---|---|---|---|---|---|---|---|---|---|---|
| | | 10 | 20 | 30 | 40 | 50 | 60 | 70 | 80 | 90 |
| % Points where first serve is in | 62.0% | | | | | X | | | | |
| % Points won when 1st serve was in | 63.0% | | X | | | | | | | |
| % Points won when a 2nd serve was required | 42.0% | | X | | | | | | | |
| % Serving points were aces | 6.8% | | | | | X | | | | |
| % Serving points were double faults | 4.9% | | | | | | | X | | |
| % Points where player went to net | 17.8% | | | | | | X | | | |
| % Net points won | 70.0% | | | | | | X | | | |
| Mean first serve speed (km.h$^{-1}$) | 185.6 | | | | | | X | | | |
| Mean second serve speed (km.h$^{-1}$) | 145.6 | | | | | | | | | X |

A further consideration is that some performance indicators cannot be considered in isolation. A player serving a relatively high number of double faults may also be serving a high number of aces and serve winners. A serve winner is where the server wins the point without playing a second shot because the opponent has failed to return the ball into court. The player may not be able to reduce the number of double faults without also reducing the number of aces and serve winners. All of these variables are related to service speed and placement.

Another example is where one player wins 70 per cent of points when the first serve is in and 50 per cent of points when relying on a second serve while the opponent wins 65 per cent of points when the first serve is in and 45 per cent of points when relying on a second serve. It appears as though the player performs better on serve than the opponent. However, if the player's first serve is only in on 40 per cent of points then the player will win 58 per cent of service points ($40 \times 70/100 + 60 \times 50/100$). If the opponent's first serve is in on 80 per cent of service points then the opponent will win 61 per cent of service points ($80 \times 65/100 + 20 \times 45/100$).

## EXAMPLES OF POOR AND GOOD PERFORMANCE INDICATORS

To sum up this section on the qualities of performance indicators, Table 3.7 shows some examples of variables (some are not even variables) that are not performance indicators. The third column of the table shows a revised variable that might be a performance indicator if all four qualities of performance indicators are met.

The colour of a team's kit may seem like a trivial example of a factor that is irrelevant to sports performance. However, there is published research claiming that kit colour may be associated with success in sport (Attrill *et al.*, 2008; Greenlees *et al.*, 2008).

There are valid performance indicators which can be used poorly by coaches. Imagine a performance indicator 'number of shots' in an invasive team game. The number of shots taken represents the ability to create scoring opportunities. However, not all shots are the same and some may be taken where there is little chance of scoring and a better tactical option might have been to play the ball to a team-mate in a better position to shoot. Consider a coach advising players that team selection would be

74

Table 3.7 Poor and better examples of performance indicators

| Not a performance indicator | Problem | Potential performance indicator |
|---|---|---|
| Net performance | This is too vague | The percentage of net points that are won (if we have a clear definition of what a net point is) |
| Whether a point is a net point | This is an action variable for a single point rather than an indicator of match performance | The percentage of net points that are won (if we have a clear definition of what a net point is) |
| Number of aces served in the match | Tennis matches have differing numbers of points meaning the value could be relatively high or low | Percentage of service points where an ace is served |
| The distance a soccer player travels dribbling the ball in a match | We do not know what range of values to expect for this variable or whether it is associated with success | The variable needs to be replaced with a variable that is understood permitting decisions to be made if we know its value |
| The percentage of match time a player spends performing high intensity activity | The variable is open to subjective judgement of movement intensity at the time of data collection | The percentage of match time a player spends running or sprinting (if we have a good definition of the distinction between jogging and running) |
| The percentage of match time a player spends moving at 4m.s$^{-1}$ or faster observed by human operator | The variable is objective but human observers could not judge the 4m.s$^{-1}$ threshold exactly. | The percentage of match time a player spends moving at 4m.s$^{-1}$ or faster recorded by an automatic player tracking system |
| Colour of team kit | Questionable validity – the variable is not relevant to coaching decision making | The analyst needs to look at more relevant areas of performance |

**sports performance data and information**

based on shots taken during a series of friendly games. Some players may decide to shoot from long distances simply to increase their number of shots. The problem here is that the players are playing to maximise their value for some performance indicator rather than playing in a way that maximises the team's chance of winning the match.

Former England goalkeeper, David James, wrote an excellent article about statistics in sport in the *Guardian* (www.theguardian.com/football/2007/dec/30/sport.comment1, accessed 4 April 2013) which included a story about a Manchester Utd goalkeeper, Peter Schmeichel, taking action to 'fiddle' his Prozone statistics. Whether the story is true or not, it is a good example of how a soccer player could do this.

> Peter Schmeichel best showed how numbers can be fiddled. Years ago there was a story going round that Schmeichel got the hump because of the introduction of Prozone, so decided to prove a point. The very next match, so the tale goes, every time the ball was down the other end, Schmeichel did sets of sprints across the edge of his area to raise his high-intensity running stats. Anyone watching probably thought: 'Oh look there's Schmeichel keeping himself warm'; but he ended up beating one of the forwards on stats for that game.

## PROCESSES OF DETERMINING PERFORMANCE INDICATORS

### Statistical methods of determining valid performance indicators

There are statistical processes for determining whether variables may be performance indicators (Choi *et al.*, 2006a/b). There are two broad statistical approaches to identifying performance indicators; comparing winning and losing performances within matches (Lorenzo *et al.*, 2010) and comparing the performances of successful and less successful performers within tournaments (Rampinini *et al.*, 2009). Large databases of performance variables can be analysed to determine which most distinguish between winning and losing performers within matches. This approach can be criticised because the performance of the losing team in a match between two elite teams may still be a high quality performance. Similarly, the performance of the winning team in a match between two lower ability teams will not be as high a quality as that of an elite team.

However, the approach also has advantages. Coaches may wish to know what it is that makes the difference in matches against similar ranked opponents. A variation of this approach considers close matches and more one sided matches separately just in case the variables that distinguish between winning and losing performances are different for the two types of match (Csataljay *et al.*, 2009; Vaz *et al.*, 2011). There are sports, such as tennis, where matches are grouped into sets and games. In these sports, it is possible for a player to win the match having won fewer points than the opponent. This is referred to as quasi-Simpson's paradox (Wright *et al.*, 2013). Matches may also involve some periods where one player is dominant and other periods where the opponent is dominant. Therefore, it might be better to identify performance indicators by analysing performances at set or game level rather than using whole match performances (Choi *et al.*, 2006a). This would allow those variables associated with successful periods within matches to be identified.

Another way of relating performance variables to the results of matches is to correlate them with outcome indicators such as the winning margin (O'Donoghue, 2002). Those variables with high absolute correlations with winning margin may be considered as potential performance indicators. This approach may be favoured in high scoring sports, such as basketball, but would not be as appropriate in lower scoring sports such as soccer.

An alternative approach is to compare the performance of successful performers and less successful performers irrespective of whether they win, draw or lose matches (Koon Tek *et al.*, 2012; Reid *et al.*, 2010). For example, we could compare the performances of the 16 teams that qualify from the pool stages of the FIFA World Cup in soccer to the performances of the 16 teams that were eliminated at the end of the pool stages. Similarly, we could compare the performances of teams that finish in the top half of a round robin league competition with those of the teams that finish in the bottom half. Not all of the performances of the successful teams will be wins and not all of the performances of the less successful teams will be losses. Performance variables can be compared between the performances of the two types of team. Any variables whose values clearly differ between the two types of team may be candidate performance indicators.

A criticism of both of the broad approaches described above (comparing winning and losing performances within matches and comparing the performances of successful and less successful performers) is that they tend to identify performance indicators related to technical effectiveness. For example in tennis, the performance variables most associated with match outcome are the percentage of points won when the first serve is in and the percentage of points won when a second serve is required (O'Donoghue, 2002). If we advise tennis coaches and players that they need to win more points on both first and second serve, they might reply 'tell us something we don't know'. They may wish to know much more information about detailed tactics that give a better chance of success than other tactics.

A further issue is that some variables are about tactics and the way that players or teams play. For example, the percentage of serves played to the left third or right thirds of the target service court could be an indication of service strategy. These variables may be determined for the deuce and advantage courts when first and second serves are played (see Table 3.4 earlier). Indeed, these may also be considered separately for matches against left and right handed opponents when it comes to interpreting values. This kind of tactical variable might not be associated with match outcome. Different service strategies might also be used by players in all regions of the World rankings. The validity of a performance indicator depends on its importance, relevance and whether coaches can use it in practice to make decisions when preparing for matches. It is important to understand the way opponents play irrespective of the success with which they employ different tactics. In this sense, tactical indicators can be valid performance indicators. The validity of tactical indicators can be assessed by comparing performers reputed by experts to use strategies.

### Non-statistical methods of identifying performance indicators

Level 5 students may not be able to access or create large enough data-bases of performance data to determine valid performance indicators when undertaking assessed work. Typically, the first coursework within a Level 5 sports performance analysis module requires the student to develop a system and use it to analyse a performance in a sport of their choice. Analysing large databases of performances is outside the scope of such coursework exercises. So students need to adopt a more feasible approach to their first coursework. The important measurement issue being addressed in the first coursework is validity. The students basically need to choose an area of a sport that is important to analyse, produce a

78

system to meet information needs in this area and apply that system. This can be done without using statistical methods of identifying performance indicators. In some cases, alternative methods of determining perform-ance indicators may be better than statistical approaches. Students may also develop a system to analyse variables in an exploratory without claiming the variables are performance indicators. There are three broad non-statistical methods of identifying variables to use in your system:

- Surveying sports performance analysis research
- Surveying coaching practice/professional literature
- Using expert opinion

There are some sports that have been researched to a greater extent than others with research evidence supporting the use of stated performance indicators. Students can critically review papers selecting performance indicators for the chosen aspect of the given sport. Students should not be worried that their own coursework appears to lack originality. They still need to devise a system to collect the necessary data to determine performance indicator values. Furthermore, the performance indicators may never have been applied at the level of the sport that the student is looking at. The student will, therefore, be producing new information about the sport at the given level.

There are other sports that have not been addressed as much in sports performance analysis research, if at all. Where the student wishes to analyse a sport of interest that has received little or no research atten-tion, they can start with professional coaching literature to identify data sources and variables. Coaching guides in the sport of interest will typi-cally identify important areas of performance, techniques involved and tactical aspects. These may be broad and vague areas when presented in some coaching guides. The student can choose one of these areas and devise operationalised variables to represent the chosen aspects of performance. In choosing aspects to look at, the student needs to make sure that there will be enough data to record to satisfy the coursework requirements but not too much data to record. In some sports, the analy-sis could be focused on a narrow area if it is repeated enough within the performance and there are several variables relating to it. In other sports, it may be necessary to analyse multiple event types to ensure there is a sufficient volume of data given the expected effort required for the coursework.

In preparing this chapter, the author decided to put himself in the position of a student wishing to analyse a sport which had received no attention to his knowledge from performance analysis research. The first thing the author did was look at the sports practice books in his university's library. The shelves were dominated by books on popular sports to an even greater extent than the author had imagined. There was a book on windsurfing (Evans, 1986) which would be a good example of a sport with little performance analysis research. A difference between the author and a student undertaking a performance analysis coursework addressing windsurfing is that the student choosing such a sport would have done so because of interest and/or experience in the sport. Hopefully, this attempt by the author, with no knowledge of windsurfing tactics or techniques, to identify areas of the sport that can be looked at will encourage readers to apply performance analysis to sports they have knowledge of and interest in.

The first thing to explore is the nature of the sport, different styles of the sport, different types of competition, rules and, very importantly, what the criteria are for winning. Evan's (1986: 132–5) book covers judging, rules, compulsory tricks in windsurfing and fixed routines. Performing tricks is a key aspect of performance in freestyle windsurfing. Types of trick that can be analysed include pirouettes, flips, jumps, splits and rail-rides. In addition to tricks, another area of performance that could be covered by an analysis system is transitions between tricks. Different types of sailing are also described by Evans (1986) including stern first and leeward sailing. The number of tricks performed, the technical difficulty of the tricks, the originality of the routine, style in execution of the tricks and style of the whole routine are judged. Each of these characteristics is reported in Evan's book as being judged out of 20 giving a total of 100. Given that the book is a 1986 book and the sport might have evolved since, the next step for the student would be to use the internet to determine current regulations for the sport. The student's system does not necessarily have to apply these regulations to produce a performance score; the purpose of the student's system may not be to judge the performance. However, it is useful to understand how the sport is judged to demonstrate the validity of any aspect of the sport chosen for analysis. Counting the number of each type of trick performed will provide some basic information which could be used to compare different performances in the student's coursework. However, the coursework would achieve a better mark if the system also analysed the quality of execution of the tricks performed. In looking for additional data to record, we can find tricks being classified as spectacular or graceful (Evans, 1986: 132). Evans (1986: 136) also recommended avoiding slipping on the board during the performance. Balance is mentioned as important when performing a rail-ride (Evans, 1986: 138–9). There are also variations of rail-rides which could be distinguished by an analysis system such as backwards and reverse rail-rides (Evans, 1986: 140–1).

In the above paragraph, only one reference has been used; the only windsurfing book in the university's library. The student should consider what aspects of windsurfing they will analyse and whether these are broadly tactical, technical or work-rate related. The student can then cover literature of how the broad aspect of performance is addressed in other sports, referring to supporting literature and establishing a rationale for applying these principles within windsurfing. The system can then be developed, applied and evaluated. So if readers wish to analyse a sport of interest, but are struggling to find literature on it, there is a way that the sport can be used in their coursework. Lecturing staff marking such coursework are always interested in work that applies sports performance analysis to new sports.

The third way of identifying variables to analyse is to use expert opinion. This can be done during exploratory interviews with individual coaches or using a focus group. An example of this was a study of Rugby World Cup performance (McCorry et al., 1996) where the two analysts were not from a rugby background. They consulted a rugby expert during an interview about areas of the game that were important. This interview was interspersed with periods of watching a video of a rugby match allowing the expert to explain important events and how they can be recognised. Students need to consider whether it will be possible to interview an expert coach within their university or an expert they have contact with outside. In a class of 100 or more sports performance analysis students, there may be 20 or more wishing to interview the university soccer coach. The coach will not be able to grant interviews to all of the students wishing to avail of his or her expertise.

Irrespective of the method used to identify areas of performance to analyse, the student should consider which variables are most important and the feasibility of collecting the raw data required. The development of a system to gather data, analyse data and present information is the subject of Chapter 4 of this book.

## SUMMARY

There is a distinction between data and information. Data are input into some process which produces resulting information. Sports performance analysis is typically a reductive approach which takes raw input performance data and summarises these in output information. There are different types of raw data that can be gathered by analysts including categorical data and numerical data. The term performance indicator is used for variables that possess certain qualities and is not a term used for all sports performance information. This chapter has listed the essential qualities that a variable must have in order to be a performance indicator. It must represent some valid and important aspect of the sport. It must have an objective measurement process. It should have a known scale of measurement. Finally, it must have a means of interpretation.

There are statistical and non-statistical processes of determining performance indicators for a sport. These have been discussed and students are encouraged to use a feasible method of identifying potential performance indicators. Literature surveys, coaching texts and expert opinion are all good ways of identifying areas of a sport for analysis. These then need to be operationalised so that a system can be created to gather the necessary data to produce information about performances.

# CHAPTER 4

## DEVELOPING ANALYSIS SYSTEMS

### INTRODUCTION

This chapter covers the lifecycle of sports performance analysis systems including the stages of requirements elicitation, system design, proto-typing, reliability testing, operation and maintenance. Requirements elicitation is a key stage of system development where the analyst and coach need to determine the key areas of performance of interest and how these can be measured. The manner in which raw data are collected to efficiently produce the desired outputs is a design matter. Typically, requirements elicitation and system design do not happen in a sequence with requirements being stabilised before design commences. Instead, an evolutionary prototyping approach sees requirements elicitation and prototype design iterated until the coach and analyst are happy with the system. System operators can then be trained to use the system and the reliability of the system can be determined using an inter-operator agreement study. The system is then used within the coaching context but may require enhancements due to rule changes, changing coaching emphasis or to exploit developments in sports analysis and feedback technology.

### THE SYSTEM LIFECYCLE

The lifecycle of a system includes its original development, application in the field and maintenance. Sports performance analysis systems are generally not decommissioned at the end of their life-time, although computer hardware that the systems run on may become obsolete. The system development process depends on a number of factors including the nature of user groups, technology available and the scale of the system. Large-scale systems involving multiple data collection and analysis processes, large databases and expensive equipment need to be developed in a similar way to large-scale computerised systems in other areas of business. Figure 4.1 is a 'V' shaped system development model used by the European space Agency (Robinson, 1992). The main characteristic that distinguishes this from the approaches used in the development of smaller-scale systems are the design stages. A large-scale system may require a team of developers. Before the implementation of components can be done, the development team need an understanding of the complete system specification, the role and purpose of any components they are developing and how these components interact with other parts of the system. The current chapter is pitched more at systems to be developed by a single analyst which involve the same stages of system development. Requirements analysis is a particularly important stage because mistakes made here might not be detected until user acceptance testing which takes place during validation of the system. Such errors require a great deal of design and implementation effort to be redone. The earlier mistakes are made, the more costly they are to correct. Therefore, requirements analysis should include acceptance test planning where customers agree the acceptance test to be used. The acceptance test can act as a means of clarifying requirements and eliciting further requirements. Once requirements have been analysed, the system can be specified in terms of input data, output information, databases and data processing functions involved. The specification describes 'what' the system will do. Verification tests whether the eventual system satisfies the specification. The difference between verification and validation is that verification tests a system to the developers' satisfaction whereas validation tests whether the system meets the users' actual requirements. When designing the system, the developers move from 'what' to the 'how'. Architectural design is carried out by senior developers who determine the overall structure of the system including the main processes, data stores and user interfaces. Detailed design ensures that those implementing individual components have a complete understanding of component functions, inputs, outputs, data structures, communication protocols and interfaces.

The principle of moving from 'what' to 'how' is not just a general system development principle, but it has also been proposed in the specific

84

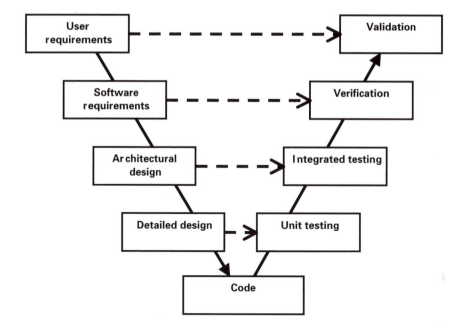

**Figure 4.1** The 'V' shaped development model for large-scale software systems

development of notation systems. Hughes and Franks (2004c: 122) stated the following:

> Unless you have a crystal-clear idea about what data you wish to collect, you will find that your system will collect confusing, and sometimes irrelevant, information.

When one considers the development process shown in Figure 4.1, a complete understanding of what is required from a system helps avoid many costly mistakes being made during system development. Coaches need to be involved as early as possible in the development of systems providing as much detail about what they require as possible. Requirements elicitation is a difficult area with user groups often providing vague and incomplete requirements for a system and expecting developers to produce an acceptable system.

The approach described above specifies the system requirements (the 'what') before devising the mechanisms to record and analyse data (the 'how'). This approach is used in large-scale system development but may also be useful in the development of smaller-scale sports performance analysis systems. Franks and Goodman (1984) listed three tasks in evaluating sports performance; describing the sport, prioritising key factors of sports performance and devising efficient data recording and analysis methods. The first two tasks consider 'what' the system needs to do while the third of these tasks deals with 'how' a system can satisfy the requirements. However, evolutionary prototyping has also been proposed for developing sports performance analysis systems (O'Donoghue and Longville, 2004) with requirements not being fully understood when implementation of system components commences. Figure 4.2 shows the evolutionary prototyping approach to develop a netball analysis system described by O'Donoghue and Longville (2004). An initial prototype was developed and used to analyse part of a game simply to show the coach what the software package (Focus X2, Elite Sports Analysis, Delgaty Bay, Fife, Scotland) was capable of. This promoted discussion with the coach and help elicit requirements for the system. The system went through a series of changes during an iterative process of implementation and requirements elicitation with the coach involved at each stage and players making suggestions that were implemented in later prototypes. One version of the system was used, synthesising the data collection process using a match video rather than a live match. This raised usability issues that were subsequently addressed. This is an example of a 'Dry run' of the system where it is tested to ensure that it works without having to analyse a full performance or use the system at a live match.

The evolutionary prototyping approach is facilitated by the fact that computerised match analysis systems are developed using generic video tagging packages with many systems being specialised versions of a general video tagging system that produces statistical output with interactive access to related video sequences. The core elements of 'player', 'position', 'action' and 'time' (Hughes and Franks, 2004b: 111) are common to many systems and experienced developers can use their knowledge of such systems to suggest requirements to users.

Irrespective of whether evolutionary prototyping, the 'V' shaped development process or some other process of system development is to be used, there are requirements analysis, system specification and testing activities to be done that are discussed in the remaining sections of the

86

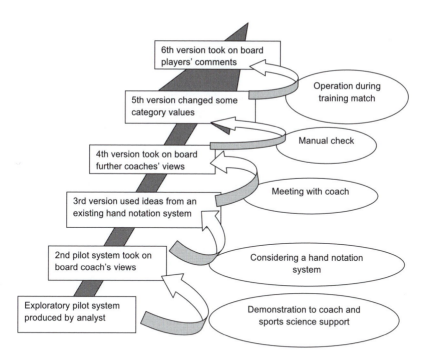

Figure 4.2 Evolutionary development of a match analysis system
(O'Donoghue and Longville, 2004)

chapter. Once the system is delivered, it needs to be maintained and regularly enhanced to incorporate new features required by coaches.

## REQUIREMENTS ANALYSIS

### Types of requirement

There are two broad types of requirements for a system; functional requirements and non-functional qualities (Pyle *et al.*, 1993: 32). Functional requirements include:

- Input data
- Output information
- Data repositories (stores) within systems
- Processes or functions
- Data flows between processes and/or data repositories as well as users

Figure 4.3 is a dataflow diagram for a semi-automatic player tracking system. The ellipses represent processes, while the trays (video frames, player trajectories, etc.) are data repositories. Data sources such as cameras as well as interaction with operators, such as quality control personnel, are also shown within the dataflow diagram. Some of the processes within the system are complicated functions that can be broken down further within lower level dataflow diagrams. Indeed, large-scale systems are often designed as a hierarchy of functions with the overall system as a single high-level process at the top of the hierarchy. Any input data need to be specified in terms of structure, volume and type of data. The input data may be event details that are entered for multiple events within matches. Each event may be characterised by the event type, outcome, player performing the event, location of the event on the playing surface and the time at which the event occurred. Event records may vary in structure depending on the event type. For example, in tennis we may wish to know the serving player, winning player, point type, number of shots and whether the point emanated from a first or second serve for all points.

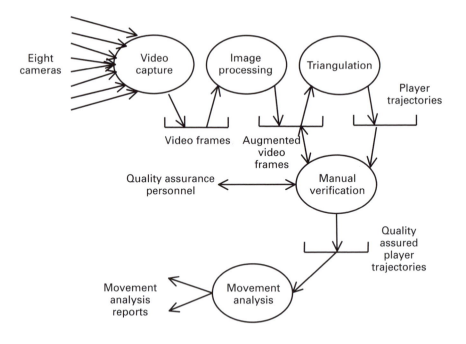

**Figure 4.3** Data flow diagram for a player tracking system

developing analysis systems

If the point type is an ace, serve winner, return winner or double fault then we do not need any additional information about the point ending. However, if the point type is a net point or baseline rally, we will need a further data item within the event record to signify whether the point ended with a winner or error. The volume, format and structure of system outputs also need to be understood. The precise layout of output information can be deferred until later in the development process, but the outputs themselves do need to be known. The system processes are functions that transform data into information. As mentioned in Chapter 3, the output of any process is information produced with respect to that process but may be input data with respect to another process. Systems often need to store video and event databases which can be analysed by interactive functions. The data repositories need to be specified including volumes and types of data. Very often systems need to be developed so that they can easily be used to answer *ad hoc* queries that had not been anticipated at the time of system development.

The dataflow diagram shows static functional requirements. There is another type of functional requirements referred to as dynamic functional requirements which are concerned with the order of system events, iterations of system actions, system states and transition between states. Figure 4.4 shows a state chart for a tennis timing system (O'Donoghue and Liddle, 1998). The system has three main states:

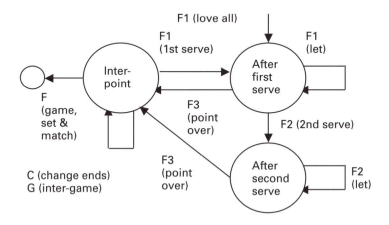

Figure 4.4 Dynamic model of a tennis match

- Between points
- Post first serve
- Post second serve

The circles in Figure 4.4 represent states which are timed. The arrows represent instantaneous events such as a serve being struck or a point ending that make the transition from one state to another. When the first serve is struck, the system cannot know whether the serve will be in or not. The timing from this point depends on the next event to be entered. If the next event is the end of the point, then the timing is for the rally. If, however, the next event is another first serve (in the case of a let) or a second serve, then the timing is for an inter-serve time. Hence the state is termed 'Post first serve'.

There are other requirements as well as those relating to the functionality of the system. These non-functional qualities are concrete constraints, system performance requirements and dependability requirements (Pyle *et al.*, 1993: 39–42). Concrete constraints include geographical location of data repositories or functions, size, weight and power consumption of equipment to be used. Battery capacities required to use the system in some environments need to be specified. The term 'performance requirements', as used here, refers to the performance of the system rather than the performance of athletes. System performance requirements are concerned with how quickly systems can perform tasks and these requirements include throughput of transactions and response time. Where event data are entered while match events are being performed, CPU (central processing unit) time is largely idle as today's computers are easily fast enough to process 1,000s of inputs during a 60-minute match. However, some systems can be set up to send a delayed video feed to an external screen on the bench for players and coaches to view after critical incidents have occurred. This video information is being produced and sent to the external screen while input video frames are being captured and the video is being tagged by the user entering events. Unless computers have fast enough CPUs, there may be dropped frames. A further consideration is that the additional processing of a delayed video feed places greater demands on the CPU and, therefore, batteries will run out quicker than if no delayed feed was produced. Therefore, system performance requirements may be related to concrete constraints. Dependability is concerned with system availability and failure during operation. Metrics such as mean time between failure and rate of failure

developing analysis systems

occurrence are used with computerised systems (Sommerville, 1992: 394–5). As well as these dependability requirements for systems and the computers they operate on, there will be recovery requirements. For example, analysts might insist on a package saving the video being captured periodically in the event of power failure or software error causing the system to crash. Dependability requirements are linked to functional requirements with respect to backup data storage.

The interface of a system can be created and changed very rapidly using the generic match analysis packages available today. This helps to promote a user-centred approach to interface development which has been recognised as essential in the development of computerised systems for almost three decades (Norman and Draper, 1986). Interfaces can be created, shown to users, pilot tested and amended within a flexible development approach.

## Viewpoint oriented requirements elicitation

Viewpoint oriented requirements elicitation involves considering the intended system from multiple perspectives including hardware constraints, usability issues, user groups, the coaching application and the role of analysts. The various viewpoints are represented by stakeholders who are consulted during the requirements analysis process. The most important viewpoint is that of the coaches who will be the ultimate end users of the system. The coach is considered to be the best technical expert from whom information needs for the system can be determined (Hughes and Franks, 2004b: 108). The coach can also represent the coaching philosophy used (Franks *et al.*, 1983) which helps identify specific information needs related to strategies used by players and teams. Franks *et al.* (1983) also described how requirements gathering can be guided by considering the primary objectives of the sport and a database of past games.

In considering the sport, abstract models of performance can be constructed and presented as flowcharts (Hughes and Franks, 2004b: 108). These flowcharts represent games as logical sequences of events (Hughes and Franks, 2004b: 109) such as alternating possessions in team games. The sequence of events that can be observed during a match follows a syntax (Olsen and Larsen, 1997) such that in some states, there are a restricted number of things that could happen in the next event.

91

These conceptual models of sports performance can be arranged into hierarchies of flowcharts (Franks and Goodman, 1984) with broad possessions and possession changes being modelled at a high level of abstraction, with possessions being broken down within more detailed models that consider how possessions commenced and ended as well as details of events within possessions. A criticism of this approach is that it could involve a possession change being entered twice. Therefore, analysts dealing with such requirements need to recognise where one team's possession ending and another team's possession commencing are the same event. For example, if a pass is intercepted, this is the end of one possession for the team that lost the ball and the beginning of another possession for the team that made the interception. The hierarchical structure shown in Figure 5.1 of Hughes and Franks' (2004b: 109) book chapter is not strictly a hierarchy. A ball possession can certainly be broken down into 'Gained' and 'Lost' as well as activity during the possession. However, the lower level information of player, specific action and location of event are data items at the same level rather than a hierarchical structure of events. Figure 4.5 shows a high-level flowchart for possessions and possession changes where possession is broken down to a lower level flow chart showing territorial information within the possession.

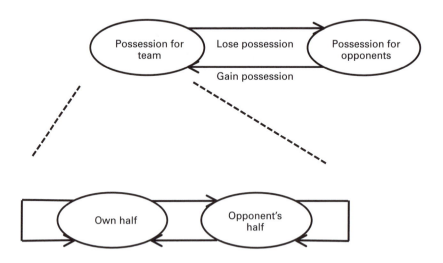

**Figure 4.5** Hierarchical model of sports behaviour

Individual events within possessions can include passes with further information about type and outcome of pass (Hughes and Franks, 2004c: 122). The number of successful and unsuccessful passes that are performed determine the percentage of passes that were successful. The coach can advise targets for such a variable, but it is important that any targets are realistic for the performer's current ability (Franks *et al.*, 1983).

Coaches in team games may advise that information is needed at team, subsidiary unit and player level (Hughes and Franks, 2004b: 113–7). Gerisch and Reicheldt (1991) have shown how the same raw information about one-on-one situations in soccer can be used to evaluate individual player as well as overall team performance.

The developers will often be the analysts themselves or people with considerable sports performance analysis experience. The developers can represent the viewpoint of the working analyst using the eventual system to analyse matches. The requirements gathered from user groups may be unfeasible. For example, there may be things the users would like to have analysed live that cannot be analysed live. For example, in a soccer match it would be impossible to enter the player making a pass, pitch location, type of pass and outcome of the pass live during a match. Similarly, user groups may require large amounts of team, opposition and individual player data to be entered post-match for a debriefing the morning after the match. In some cases, this may not be possible for the analyst. Developers need to consider the requirements made by user groups and calculate the rate of event entry for live systems and the volume of time required for post-match analysis. These will be estimates, but it is possible to analyse a small portion of a match video to improve the accuracy of such estimates. Event rates are used when considering live systems because there is a pre-set time equal to the match time with events having to be entered as they occur. Post-match analysis is not limited to match time and so the volume of work is expressed in terms of hours required.

Other viewpoints to be considered include ergonomic issues to do with viewing position, physical environment of analysis tasks and human-computer interface. Sports performance analysis systems have followed advances in input and output peripheral devices over the years (Hughes and Franks, 1995). Digitisation tablets (Dufour, 1991), voice-over input (Taylor and Hughes, 1988; Cort, 2006), graphical user interfaces (Hughes and Franks, 2004a: 103) and touch sensitive screens (Claudio and Dimas, 1995) have all been used as input devices for match analysis systems.

While the graphical user interface is a technological advance over the traditional keyboard, keyboard interfaces may be more accurate for the collection of match event data. This is because the user needs to operate a mouse as well as check the location of the match pointer on screen when using a graphical user interface. This might not hold for all analysis tasks for all sports and so analysts need to consider the relative merits of different input methods for the given task. There are also automated and semi-automated methods of gathering data such as GPS devices (Carling *et al.*, 2008; Carling and Bloomfield, 2013) and ultra-wide band (UWB) radio signals (Leser and Kwon, 2014).

The capacity of hardware needs to be considered. This viewpoint covers battery capacity under different modes of operation, video capture and processing capability and wireless communication possibilities. Time needed for video compression or producing DVDs or video outputs on other devices needs to be considered as these tasks delay other tasks while the analyst's machine is in use. Computer batteries last for different amounts of time depending on disk and processor usage. Some analysts have to dim their computer screen when operating under battery power to ensure the battery lasts for the full match.

There may be conflicting requirements coming from different viewpoints, particularly between what the users require and what analysts operating the system are capable of. Such conflicts need to be discussed and resolved during requirements analysis. One way of doing this is to arrange viewpoints into a hierarchy so that there is a higher order viewpoint represented, the stakeholder of which can arbitrate in such cases (Curran *et al.*, 1994).

## SYSTEM DESIGN AND IMPLEMENTATION

Design and implementation activities can either be done after requirements are understood and the system is specified or they can be done intermittently during an evolutionary prototyping approach that alternates these activities with requirements analysis. Design and implementation are about devising methods of achieving system aims. The difference between design and implementation is that implementation develops a prototype or final system on the intended hardware/software platform while design devises methods at a more abstract level prior to implementation. In evolutionary prototyping approaches, there will be design activity during early proto-

94

type development but once the broad solution of functions, inputs, outputs and data stores is understood, the evolutionary prototyping approach typically alternates requirements and implementation activities. Design and implementation stages involve pen and paper when dealing with manual notation systems. Of course, prototype and final system forms can be word processed and printed out. The distinction between design and implementation stages for manual notation systems is that design activities consider systems macroscopically identifying where forms are used to capture, store or process data as well as the output forms to be used. The implementation of a manual notation system is the actual development of the form rather than merely identify that there will be a particular form.

When implementing systems, developers should ensure that data collection and analysis are as simple as possible (Hughes and Franks, 2004c: 128). There will be many possible methods of achieving the same result and developers need to consider feasible alternatives in terms of their usability in the analysis environment. The data recording tasks should reflect the order of events within the sport so that data recording becomes an extension of the observation task. Capturing two pieces of information in the order they are observed (A then B) can dramatically improve the usability of the system. Even though entering B then A requires the same volume of data gathering, the analyst needs to view the game in an unnatural way remembering the event A so that it can be entered after B. An example of this is when entering the cause and then outcome of a tennis player approaching the net (O'Donoghue, 2010: 140–1). A pilot version where outcome of a net point was entered before the cause of approaching the net was quite awkward to use in comparison.

When developing computerised systems, the placement of buttons on graphical user interfaces needs to consider the order of information being entered by the analyst. A simple arrangement of button clusters can allow simple left to right movement of the cursor (mouse pointer) during data entry for a given event. There are also 'activation links' in some systems that initiate higher order events automatically when a lower order event is entered. This can cut down on the volume of data entry activity required by the analyst. A further possibility is the use of scripts to process the data that have been entered in order to automatically produce higher order information (O'Donoghue, 2013a). This does require very skilled developers as not all analysts can program scripts. Fortunately programming a script can be done during system development and does not need to be repeated each time the final system is used.

A system can be used to successfully enter data and analyse that data but outputs may be ineffective due to poor presentation. In other words, the system satisfies its functional requirements and provides the correct output information but it is in a form that fails to convey the information effectively. Hughes and Franks (2004c: 132) stated that the whole system will be judged on its outputs which need to be clear, well laid out and presented simply. Chapters 5 and 6 will go into detail on form design and outputs for manual notation systems while Chapters 7 and 8 will cover the layout of data entry screens in computerised systems as well as output screens.

## SYSTEM TESTING

Before systems are applied in the field, they need to be tested to ensure that they are usable and work correctly. Testing activity does not need to wait until a system is completed, especially if the system is a large-scale system involving multiple computerised components and operators. Testing does not always need to be applied to a whole match as a system can be tested using a short period of the match (Hughes and Franks, 2004c: 128). There are different types of testing activity that can be done during system development. These include:

- Module testing
- Integrated testing
- Usability testing
- Verification
- Reliability testing
- Validation

Module testing involves testing whether a system component works correctly. For example, an input component can be tested to ensure that match data is created as intended. In sportscode (Sportstec, Warriewood, New South Wales, Australia), a code window is used to enter events into a timeline. Some events have specified lead and lag times which need to be checked to ensure that video sequences for those events include all of the action that coaches and players would need to see to discuss the causes and consequences of events. Developers should check that all exclusive links work as intended with events terminating any other events they are exclusively linked to. Similarly, activation links should be checked to determine that events activate other events that they are required to automatically trigger.

Output components need to be tested to ensure that they display the correct information for the given raw data that have been recorded. In evolutionary prototyping, the input components and any processing components would be developed before output components. The system should be tested as each component is added. This is because errors made in an input component can lead to propagation errors within processing and output components. There may be situations where it is necessary to develop an output component prior to input and processing components in order to facilitate discussion with user groups about system requirements. In situations like this, the developers need to synthesise any components that the output component uses. For example, in sports-code the developers might produce a statistics window that simply contains test values that are sent to output components without any programming of scripts to produce such values from input data.

Integrated testing is where multiple components are tested to ensure they work together. Where an evolutionary prototyping approach is used, integrated testing happens as new components are added to the evolving system. This is an example of 'bottom-up' development where the system is designed as a hierarchy of processes but implementation is done with the lower level components being completed first. 'Top-down' implementation is possible where high-level components can be tested using dummy lower level components rather than the completed actual components they need to invoke.

Usability testing is particularly important for systems with intensive human operated components. The demands that data entry tasks place on system operators may not be fully understood until such activities are tested. It may turn out that, while a software system can be developed to record match data, it is not possible for a human operator to enter these data live while observing a match. This means that alternative design solutions will need to be considered with some area of data entry being delayed until post-match analysis. Users become more competent at operating systems with practice and, therefore, a user interface should not be dismissed as inoperable until sufficient testing has been done. Usability testing should also be done as early as possible to avoid a lot of unnecessary system development activity where input components are too difficult to use.

Once a system is completed, no matter whether it is a manual or computerised system, it needs to be assessed for reliability. The computerised part of a system may be deterministic, but the human component of the system may be prone to error. Inter-operator reliability studies are used to determine the objectivity of a system. Two operators analyse the same performance(s) using the system independently. Any disagreements between the operators represent limitations in the reliability of the system which may be minor or major concerns to user groups. Reliability is discussed in more detail in Chapter 9.

Verification involves testing the entire system to ensure it works as the developers intended while validation tests that the system actually fulfils the needs of the user groups.

## OPERATION AND MAINTENANCE

Once a system is completed, it can be used within coaching or whatever other application area it was intended for. However, systems rarely stay the same for very long and need to be enhanced for various reasons. There may be further information needed by coaches that was not in the original system. This could be because of coaching staff changing or team tactics requiring specific information to be analysed. Systems also need to be revised to follow advances in feedback technology. The author developed a netball analysis system in the Focus X2 package in 2004 which has undergone many changes in the years since. One change was to split a broad turnover event into different types of turnover. Another issue was that there were matches involving future opponents where filming was not permitted. Therefore, a manual version of the system was developed to allow the same statistics to be determined for the future opponents as for the author's own team. After the system had been used for two seasons, it was possible to develop norms for different performance variables to help interpret performances in future matches. When the author moved with the coach to another squad where Apple Macintosh machines were used instead of IBM PC compatible computers, it was necessary to implement the system in sportscode. The main issue here was that Focus X2 abstracts behaviour to instantaneous events whereas sportscode can also abstract behaviour to events that have a non-zero duration. The sportscode package also allowed a statistics window to produce automatic outputs during the match. Further developments

98

have seen the system used to provide video sequences to players on internet based packages such as Team Performance Exchange (Team Performance Exchange, Best, Netherlands) and Replay (Replay Analysis, London, UK). Wireless communication through airport boxes allows data to be sent to iPhones and iPads which can be used by coaches on the bench to report to players during intervals between match periods. These progressions in feedback technology have also facilitated fundamental changes in the coaching process itself which can lead to other information needs emerging.

Rule changes in sports also require systems to change. For example, the challenge system in tennis means that data entered for a point that has been played may need to change as a result of the challenge made. A system developed by the author (O'Donoghue and Ingram, 2001) would not be able to be used today because the system saves the data entered for a point as soon as the point ends prior to a challenge being made. Therefore, if the system was to be used today, it would need to be enhanced to allow a point record to be changed as a result of a challenge being made. This would need to be implemented in a way that was simple and effective without being cumbersome to operate.

## SUMMARY

The lifespan of a system includes its development and period of operation in the field. The most important stage of system development is requirements analysis because it is necessary to produce a system that fulfils the users' actual needs. The process of system development depends on the type and size of the system. Large-scale systems need structured designs to provide an understanding of the overall system allowing individual developers to proceed with the development of components. Smaller-scale systems are typically developed using an evolutionary prototyping approach. System testing should be carried out frequently during the development of a system with integrated testing being done as new components are added. Systems involving a human operator component need to be assessed for reliability. As rules change and coaching requirements change, systems need to be enhanced to meet changing information needs. Furthermore, systems should be upgraded to take advantage of technological developments that are beneficial to feedback within the coaching process.

# CHAPTER 5

## GUIDELINES FOR MANUAL NOTATION SYSTEMS

### INTRODUCTION

This chapter goes into the detail of designing manual notation systems. During system design, the analyst must consider the raw data to be collected, what has to be observed, the resulting information format and decisions that are going to be made by coaches. What is the most efficient way of recording the required raw data? What is the most efficient way of recording raw data to allow resulting outputs to be produced? Is it necessary to use a scatter chart, a chronological event list or is a tallying system appropriate? Guidelines are given on when to use each type of system, form design and layout.

### WHY USE MANUAL NOTATION?

Today, there are cost effective computerised video analysis systems which can be tailored for use in different sports. Some of these systems are useful for analysing technique while others are better for analysing broader tactical aspects of game sports. General purpose data processing packages such as Microsoft Excel and database packages such as Microsoft Access can also be set up to provide user-friendly data entry interfaces as well as data structures that are suitable for rapid processing by the computer. In the case of Microsoft Excel, a Visual BASIC front end can be used, for example. An analyst could be quite a wizard at using all of the packages mentioned above but might not necessarily be a good performance analyst. Professor Mike Hughes once commented to the

# 100

author about a group of students that the author was concerned about who were working away with one of the video analysis packages 'they are good performance analysis technicians but they are not good performance analysts'. In designing the Level 5 module that the students do in the second year of their degree programmes, the staff at Cardiff Metropolitan University have intentionally used manual notation in the first half of the module before the students get hands-on experience of the software packages in the second half. Developing a manual notation system is a useful exercise for students learning sports performance analysis. The process of developing such a system requires the student to understand the sport of interest, the important aspects of the sport, operationalise these, identify raw data needed and to be able to devise a system to gather and analyse these data. Chapter 3 has covered different types of data and information used in sports performance analysis and Chapter 4 has described how these should be considered during system development. Specifically, functional requirements deal with information to be produced by a system, data to be collected and stored and the system processes that transform data into information. Hierarchical models and flowcharts can be used as abstract representations of important aspects of the sport of interest. Once we have developed a good understanding of what the system needs to do and the data and information involved, we are in a good position to develop a system. This does apply to both manual and computerised systems and so some readers may still be asking why are we covering manual notation. During the development of the system, pilot work helps to ensure that the system works as intended. It is so easy to amend input interfaces in the flexible general purpose video analysis systems we have today, that such amendments can be made without much thought. Replacing one version of a manual data collection form with another version is not so straightforward, even when it has been word-processed. This means that students developing manual notation systems will have put more thought into initial design and when amending the system during pilot work.

## TYPES OF MANUAL NOTATION SYSTEM

Hughes and Franks (2004c: 118) described three different types of manual notation form which can be used in isolation or in combination within a system. These are:

- Scatter diagrams
- Frequency tables
- Sequential systems

Examples of these manual data collection forms will be discussed in this chapter, covering different sport types and different aspects of sports performance. Scatter diagrams represent the playing surface (pitch, court, etc.) allowing the location of events of interest to be recorded. The advantages of scatter diagrams are that they allow precise locations of events to be recorded and they can be inspected by coaches very quickly during or after performances. A disadvantage of scatter diagrams is that timing and temporal information is typically not recorded. It is possible, that events could be numbered as they occur to provide such information but recording this additional data makes the scatter diagram more difficult to use.

Frequency tables are used to record tallies of events. Tallies can be recorded for combinations of event types and other variables of interest such as outcome of events. For example, a tally system could have an area to record successful and unsuccessful applications of each event type. Such a system could further be expanded to record tallies for events performed in different areas of the playing surface. In fact, whatever other variables associated with events that information is required for can be incorporated into a tally system. The advantage of a frequency table is that event frequencies are available during and shortly after performances. Where successful and unsuccessful applications of events have been tallied, it may be necessary to calculate the percentage of events performed successfully and record this on the form. This could take some minutes at the end of a match period and at the end of the match. One disadvantage of frequency tables is that precise locations of events are not recorded and we are restricted to frequencies for broad areas of the playing surface. Another disadvantage is that the chronological order of events is not recorded and we simply have totals presented in the tables.

Sequential systems record a chronologically ordered list of match events. For each event, a number of variables can be recorded such as area of the event type, playing surface, team and player performing the event and outcome of the event. The advantage of sequential systems is that they preserve the chronological order of events allowing temporal aspects of performance to be analysed. The main disadvantage of sequential systems is that further processing of data is necessary in order to determine frequency and percentage data which are not readily available once data collection has been completed. Another disadvantage of sequential systems is that precise locations of events are not recorded although broad zones where events occurred can be recorded.

## EXAMPLES OF SCATTER DIAGRAMS

### Feed analysis in netball

In netball, players are restricted to particular areas of the court. For example, the shooting circle (it is actually a semi-circle) can only be entered by the Goal Attack (GA) and Goal Shooter (GS) of the attacking team and the Goal Keeper (GK) and Goal Defender (GD) of the defending team. An important aspect of netball performance is feeding the players in the shooting circle; this is basically a pass from outside the shooting circle to inside the shooting circle. Passing may be easier outside the shooting circle because four players are allowed to play in the part of the attacking third that excludes the shooting circle; the Centre (C), Wing Attack (WA), GA and GS. Five players are allowed to play in the middle third; GD, Wing Defender (WD), C, WA and GA. When feeding, there is a maximum of two players who could receive the pass in the circle; GA and GS. Figure 5.1 shows a court diagram (scatter diagram) showing two-thirds of the court; the middle third and one attacking third. Passes can only be made within a third or between two adjacent thirds. Therefore, passes cannot be made directly from the defending third to the attacking third. This is why the defending third does not need to be shown when we are considering feeds to the shooting circle.

On the court diagram, the feeding player is shown (GD, WA, C or GA). This diagram would be for one team in one-quarter of the match. Any more data than this would obscure patterns. There is one case where a feed is notated within the shooting circle. Is this an error or not? It depends on our definition of a feed. According to the definition given here about feeding the players in the shooting circle from outside, it is an error. Other coaches may decide they wish to see the last pass before a shot is taken. In such a situation, showing the pass within the shooting circle is not an error. A further consideration with this pass shown inside the shooting circle is whether we show the feed that played the ball into the shooting circle prior to the pass. Furthermore, there are

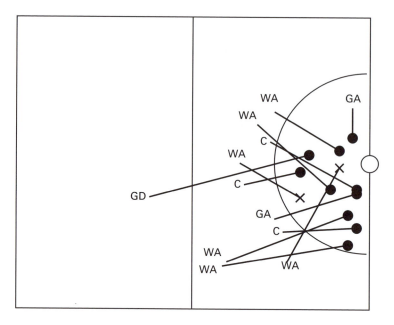

**Figure 5.1** Netball feed analysis

occasions where a player may be contacted within the shooting circle and is awarded a free pass within the circle. Thus a feed would not have been required to get the ball to a player in the shooting circle.

Each line represents the path taken by a pass without any information about pace or trajectory of the pass or whether it bounced on the court surface between the passing player and the receiving player. The symbol at the end of the line represents the outcome of the shot taken; the closed circle represents a goal and the cross represents a miss. Another issue to consider is that when a feed is made, the GS or GA can pass the ball back out of the circle if they need to find a better shooting location to receive the ball in. If we record such feeds, we may need a third outcome to represent the ball being passed back out of the circle. The best way to consider all of these issues is to watch a quarter of a netball game noting any aspects of play that need to be addressed within the system. One thing that has not been distinguished in this form is the shooting player (GA or GS). Separate sheets could be used for each shooting player in each quarter. A disadvantage of the scatter diagrams is that broad areas have not been noted, meaning statistical information is not shown on the

104

form. This statistical information can be produced by further analysing the data. However, the detail of actual location might be more beneficial to a coach and players who are looking at such a diagram as this method loses less information than a tallying approach.

## Work rate analysis in badminton

Time-motion analysis can now be done with GPS or other player tracking equipment. However, there is still a role for manual methods in analysing agility requirements, jumps and turns (Bloomfield *et al.*, 2007). Students should not be put off doing a time-motion study for coursework on manual notation but they should provide a good justification for doing so. This is because time-motion analysis is considered to be of lower importance within coaching than tactical analysis and technique analysis. The effort of producing time-motion information might not be justified by the usefulness of the information. However, there may be interesting things to analyse using manual time-motion analysis. This section describes the method used by Liddle *et al.* (1996) to compare distance covered men's singles and doubles badminton. In the absence of a computerised system, the use of video equipment was combined with hand notation of movement within rallies. A separate court diagram (a variation of a scatter diagram), such as the one shown in Figure 5.2, was used for each rally. The court diagram only shows the player's side of the court. The distance covered by a player within a rally was measured by drawing the path travelled onto the court diagram during post-match analysis. The video was paused each time the player changed direction and a line representing the phase of movement performed up to the paused video frame was drawn. A ruler was used to measure the length of path travelled. The court diagram was drawn to scale and the grid represented the 0.5m × 0.5m divisions. These 0.5m areas were shown on the video because tape was used to mark them on the side and back of the actual court. Figure 5.2 shows a court diagram completed for a rally. This is quite a paper intensive method. Once all of the rallies were analysed in this way, the distribution of rally lengths were determined. For example, a column chart could show the number or percentage of rallies where less than 5m, 5m to less than 10m, 10m to less than 15m, 15m to less than 20m, 20m to less than 25m, 25m to less than 30m and 30m or greater is covered. Supporting summary statistics such as the mean or median rally length can also be used.

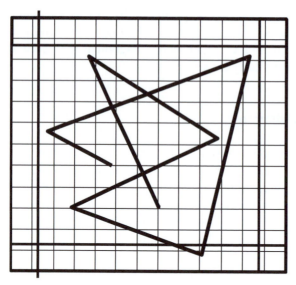

**Figure 5.2** Manual time-motion analysis of badminton (Liddle *et al.*, 1996)

## EXAMPLES OF FREQUENCY TABLES

### Passing in a team game

In team games, one of the methods of characterising the strategy of a team is by analysing the number of passes made per possession. If the mean number of passes per possession is low, the team may be adopting a direct style of play using long passes to the attackers. Where the mean number of passes per possession is high, the team may be using a more elaborate slow build-up style. Figure 5.3 shows a form used to tally possessions of different numbers of passes. The outcome of a possession is classified according to whether the ball reached the attacking third and, if it did, whether there was an opportunity to score or not. Every time the team has possession, the analyst counts the number of passes and notes the outcome before adding to the frequency being tallied in the appropriate cell. The last row (11+ passes per possession) can be used in two ways. First, it can be a row of simple tallies like the other rows. This means that calculation of the mean passes per possession is not possible due to missing information. However, the median number of passes per possession could be determined. The median possession is the one in the

106

| Passes per possession | Not entering attacking third | Enter attacking third, no attempt | Attempt off target | Attempt on target | Goal | Total |
|---|---|---|---|---|---|---|
| 1 | ⅢⅡ IIII | I | | | | 10 |
| 2 | ⅢⅡ ⅢⅡ II | I | | II | | 15 |
| 3 | ⅢⅡ ⅢⅡ ⅢⅡ | I | | | | 16 |
| 4 | ⅢⅡ ⅢⅡ II | III | | | | 15 |
| 5 | ⅢⅡ I | II | | I | I | 10 |
| 6 | III | I | II | I | | 7 |
| 7 | III | I | | | | 4 |
| 8 | I | | I | | | 2 |
| 9 | | I | | | | 1 |
| 10 | | | | | | 0 |
| 11+ | 12  13 | 15  11 | | | 12 | 5 |
| Total | 63 | 13 | 3 | 4 | 2 | 85 |

**Figure 5.3** Passes per possession

middle if the possessions are looked at in order of passes per possession. So we would determine the row totals, add these up to give a total number of possessions, N. If N is an odd number, then the median possession is possession (N+1)/2. That is if N is 85, then the median is the 43rd possession when they are considered in ascending order of passes per possession. If there are 10 possessions of one pass, 15 possessions of two passes, 16 possessions of three passes and 15 possessions of four passes, as shown in Figure 5.3, then the median is four passes. This is because the cumulative frequency for possessions of three passes or fewer is 41 and the cumulative frequency for possessions of four passes or fewer is 56. So the 43rd possession has four passes when they are considered in ascending order of passes per possession. To determine the mean, we would need to write in the number of passes per possession for each possession with 11 or more passes. For example, there might be five such possessions with 12, 15, 11, 13 and 12 passes. Imagine that we had 85 possessions as shown in Figure 5.3. The frequencies can be used to determine the mean using equation (5.1). Note that the sum uses 15 terms because we have one possession of 15 passes. In this case, the mean number of passes per possession is $(1 \times 10 + 2 \times 15 + 3 \times 16 + 4 \times 15 +$

$5 \times 10 + 6 \times 7 + 7 \times 4 + 8 \times 2 + 9 \times 1 + 10 \times 0 + 11 \times 1 + 12 \times 2 + 13 \times 1 + 14 \times 0 + 15 \times 1)/85 = 356/85 = 4.19.$

$$\text{Mean} = (\Sigma_{i=1..15} \; i \times \text{Freq}_i)/N \qquad\qquad (5.1)$$

The mean or median alone do not fully represent the team's possessions. Therefore, the data should be presented as a table or chart (Figure 5.4). This chart is a compound column chart showing the breakdown of outcomes for possessions of different numbers of passes. Hughes and Franks (2005) have shown that if scoring opportunities or goals are considered alone, we may misinterpret data. For example, in Figure 5.3 we might conclude that the most effective possessions have five or six passes because five of the nine scoring opportunities come from such possessions. However, as Hughes and Franks (2005) have explained, we also need to consider how many possessions there were of different numbers of passes to determine how productive each type is. The most effective possessions in terms of percentage entering the attacking third (including scoring opportunities) and the percentage leading to any kind of scoring opportunity (given by the last three columns) should be determined to identify the most effective possession lengths. The data shown in Figure 5.3 suggest that possessions of 11 or more passes are the most effective for entering the attacking third; 60 per cent of these possessions (3/5) resulted in the team entering the attacking third. This does exclude possessions of nine passes because there was only one of these, so either 0 per cent or 100 per cent of this one possession would have reached the attacking third. If creating a scoring opportunity is our criterion for success, then possessions of six passes are the most effective; 42.9 per cent of these possessions (3/7) resulted in a scoring opportunity. Separate forms like Figure 5.3 can be used to compare the two teams within a match. One thing students need to be aware of when describing their results is that not all possessions end when the team intended. A team may only make three passes in a particular possession because they lost possession prematurely. So the number of passes in the possession did not reflect the tactics adopted.

There are other types of passing analysis systems that could be used. For example, we could classify passes by their length (short or long), direction (forwards, backwards, left or right) and outcome (successfully completed or not). These variables would need to be defined to allow consistent analysis. For example, we could use 90° sectors as shown in

# 108

manual notation systems

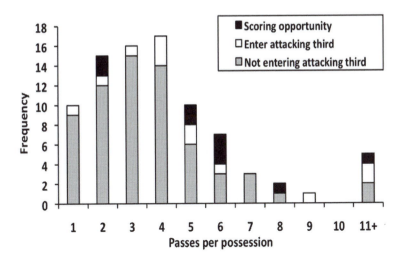

Figure 5.4 Column chart summarising effectiveness of possessions of different lengths

Figure 5.5 to classify the direction of a pass. A threshold value such as 10m could be used to distinguish between short and long passes. A successful pass is one that is received by a team-mate.

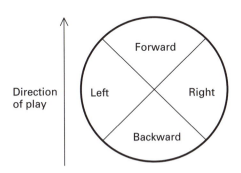

Figure 5.5 Direction of passes

**McCorry *et al.*'s (1996) rugby union system**

This example of a frequency table is about rugby union and is included as an example of developing a system to analyse territorial aspects of games and possession changes. Another reason for including it is that it was a system developed by two inexperienced analysts, including the author at the time, from non-rugby backgrounds (McCorry *et al.*, 1996). This system, therefore, serves as an example of what many students may need to do to develop a manual notation system. The analysts discussed the important aspects of rugby union with a rugby expert who advised on two broad areas for analysis. The first of these was gaining territory by entering the attacking third of the field. Methods of gaining territory irrespective of whether a team entered the attacking third were also deemed important. The second aspect was changes of possession during set play and open play.

McCorry *et al.* (1996) used an exploratory method involving several types of data collection form which eventually allowed data to be summarised. Some data that were gathered were more detailed than required. This is an example of an exploratory system where the analysts were not so familiar with information needs. Hunter and O'Donoghue (2001) used a more streamlined approach based on the known information needs for their particular study. Figure 5.6 shows a single form that could be used to gather the data required. The first two sections record whether play entered the attacking third because of poor defensive play by the defending team or good attacking play by the attacking team. McCorry *et al.* (1996) have provided examples of these. Play exits the attacking third through good defensive play, poor attacking play or because points have been scored. Methods of gaining territory, in general, are classified as around (running and passing play), over (kicking the ball forward) or through (driving, rucking and mauling) the opponents. Possession changes through open and set play are also recorded. In each type of analysis, simple tallying is used.

**Opportunity and risk**

Figure 5.7 shows a general system for analysing the opportunity and risk associated with options that sports performers have in different situations. Consider Situation 1. In this situation, Option 1a is a low risk

| Date: | |
|---|---|
| Tournament: | |
| Team A: | |
| Team B: | |
| Other information: | |

| Attacking third analysis (Team A attacking) | |
|---|---|
| Entry | Exit |
| −ve Defence (Team B)<br>Tally: | +ve Defence (Team B)<br>Tally: |
| +ve Offence (Team A)<br>Tally: | −ve Offence (Team A)<br>Tally: |
| | Scores (Team A)<br>Tally: |

| Attacking third analysis (Team B attacking) | |
|---|---|
| Entry | Exit |
| −ve Defence (Team A)<br>Tally: | +ve Defence (Team A)<br>Tally: |
| +ve Offence (Team B)<br>Tally: | −ve Offence (Team B)<br>Tally: |
| | Scores (Team B)<br>Tally: |

| Methods of gaining territory | | | | | |
|---|---|---|---|---|---|
| Team A | | | Team B | | |
| Around | Over | Around | Over | Around | Over |
| Tally: | Tally: | Tally: | Tally: | Tally: | Tally: |

| Possession changes | | | |
|---|---|---|---|
| From Team A to Team B | | From Team B to Team A | |
| Set play | Open play | Set play | Open play |
| Tally: | Tally: | Tally: | Tally: |

**Figure 5.6** Rugby analysis form

| Situation | Option | Point conceded | Worse situation | Similar situation | Better situation | Point scored |
|---|---|---|---|---|---|---|
| Situation 1 | Option 1a | | I |卌 I | II | |
| | Option 1b | | III | 卌 IIII | 卌 I | I |
| | Option 1c | II | II | II | III | I |
| Situation 2 | Option 2a | | | II | II | I |
| | Option 2b | | I | II | | I |
| | Option 2c | | | III | I | |
| Situation 3 | Option 3a | | III | I | | |
| | Option 3b | | I | 卌 | II | |
| | Option 3c | | | II | II | |
| Situation 4 | Option 4a | | I | | | |
| | Option 4b | | III | I | I | |
| | Option 4c | I | II | | | |

**Figure 5.7** Frequency table to analyse opportunity and risk of different options

option where the performer is unlikely to concede a point but also unlikely to score a point. Option 1c, on the other hand, appears to be a high risk option which could result in points being scored or conceded. There are examples of sports where the tactical choices with the highest opportunity of success also come with the highest risks (Hibbs and O'Donoghue, 2013). For example, in tennis attempting to serve an ace on second serve risks serving a double fault. There are other useful pieces of information which can be derived from Figure 5.7. For example, the performer needs to avoid getting into Situation 4 as this seems to be the start of a downward spiral leading to conceding a point with little opportunity to get to a safer state. Situation 2 is a critically important state for the performer to get into because it appears to have the greatest chance of leading to more advantageous states, especially if Option 2a is chosen in this state. In Situation 3, the performer chooses Option 3b more than any other. This option seems relatively safe. Based on the analysis done here, the performer should be advised to choose Option 3c more and to avoid Option 3a in this situation. This type of system could be tailored for use with different sports where there are different states of performance where performers have different tactical choices and these options come with differing opportunities and risks.

## EXAMPLES OF SEQUENTIAL SYSTEMS

### Middle-distance running

Middle-distance running events include the 800m and 1500m which often involve tactical use of pacing, especially in championships where athletes have to run heats, semi-finals and a final (Brown, 2005). Tactics can be evaluated using split times as well as categorical data about athlete location at different points in the race. Brown and O'Donoghue (2006) showed an example of a manual notation form (Figure 5.8) allowing the location of athletes to be recorded pictorially every 100m. This is a scatter diagram except for a track section rather than a court or pitch used in a game sport. This requires race videos to be paused at the points in the race where the athletes' locations are to be recorded. The series of images at each 100m point (for example) allows tactical assessment to be made by coaches. An alternative approach of categorising athlete location will be easier to record but still cannot be done live due to the number of athletes competing in the race. There are typically eight athletes in an 800m race and 12 athletes in a 1500m race. The 'front to back' location within the field the field of athletes can be classified as:

- Leading
- Being in the middle of the leading group
- Being at the back of the leading group
- Not being in the leading group.

The lateral location within the field of athletes can be classified as:

- Alone on the inside
- Outside a group of athletes
- Inside a group of athletes.

Using categorical variables like these, cuts down on data recording but also involves information loss compared with the pictorial approach. For example, where an athlete is on the inside of a group of athletes, they may be 'boxed in' but this depends on whether there are athletes in front of them, whether there are athletes directly behind them and how far the athlete has to go in the race. Athletes' tactics can be assessed by their location within a field of athletes at various points of the race. An athlete, running at the back of the leading pack for the first lap of an 800m before

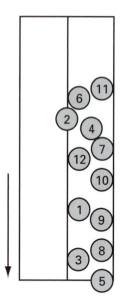

**Figure 5.8** Recording of placing and positioning data in middle distance running

moving through the field in the second lap is using different running tactics from the athlete who leads the race during the first lap. These tactical differences can be recognised using the categorical location variables or the pictorial approach. Horwill (1991) classified runners according to their tactics as leaders, pacers, breakers or kickers. It is possible that the same athlete might adopt a 'last 200m kick' tactic in some races and a 'leading' tactic in other races depending on the relative strengths and weaknesses of opponents. A major question with this type of analysis is whether it is useful? Students need to reflect on systems they are producing and ask whether they are needed. For example, a full video of an 800m race can be observed in about two minutes, so what purpose does the type of data shown in Figure 5.8 serve? Can it assist the viewing of the video if coaches and athletes know what to look for in the video? These are questions the students should ask and make a case for the analysis done when writing up coursework on it.

Split times can also be used to assess running tactics allowing athletes who run fast sections early, late or in the middle of races to be recognised. Split times are derived from elapsed times which are best analysed by directly entering them into a spreadsheet programmed in a package like

Microsoft Excel. Therefore, the system is not really a hand notation system but a special purpose computerised system is not used either. A system based on split times could be used live for a single athlete whose split times are recorded on a stopwatch or mobile phone. The system cannot be used live where multiple athletes are being analysed. Therefore, a race video has to be analysed recording the times at which athletes reach each 100m point in the race. This could be done using a stopwatch, mobile phone or painstakingly positioning the video to record the frame at which each athlete reaches each 100m point. There is a time versus accuracy trade off in choosing any of these data collection methods. The elapsed times for each athlete are entered into a spreadsheet which determines split times by subtraction. Specifically, the split time for the 100m section between 300m and 400m, for example, is the elapsed time at 400m less the elapsed time at 300m. Because some athletes are faster than others, raw split times are problematic and may be more about the fitness of the athlete than tactical aspects. Therefore, it is better to program the spreadsheet to relate split times to average split time (how much faster or slower they are than average in the race) or to relate split times to an expected split time based on the athlete's personal best time. Figure 5.9 shows an example of such a spreadsheet; the elapsed times are entered while the split times and percentage of personal best (%PB) are calculated within programmed cells. The %PB assumes an even

|        | Athlete 1 | | | Athlete 2 | | | ... | Athlete 8 | | |
|--------|------|------|-------|-------|------|-------|-----|-------|------|-------|
|        | ET   | ST   | %PB   | ET    | ST   | %PB   | ... | ET    | ST   | %PB   |
| 100m   | 14.2 | 14.2 | 98.8  | 14.3  | 14.3 | 97.4  | ... | 14.6  | 14.6 | 103.6 |
| 200m   | 28.7 | 14.5 | 100.9 | 28.8  | 14.5 | 98.7  | ... | 29.2  | 14.6 | 103.6 |
| 300m   | 43.4 | 14.7 | 102.3 | 43.6  | 14.8 | 100.8 | ... | 43.9  | 14.7 | 104.3 |
| 400m   | 57.9 | 14.5 | 100.9 | 58.3  | 14.7 | 100.1 | ... | 58.3  | 14.4 | 102.2 |
| 500m   | 72.6 | 14.7 | 102.3 | 73.3  | 15.0 | 102.1 | ... | 72.8  | 14.5 | 102.9 |
| 600m   | 87.3 | 14.7 | 102.3 | 88.5  | 15.2 | 103.5 | ... | 87.4  | 14.6 | 103.6 |
| 700m   | 102.1| 14.8 | 103.0 | 104.1 | 15.6 | 106.2 | ... | 102.1 | 14.7 | 104.3 |
| 800m   | 116.7| 14.6 | 101.6 | 119.6 | 15.5 | 105.5 | ... | 116.3 | 14.2 | 100.8 |
| PB     | 115.0|      |       | 117.5 |      |       | ... | 112.7 |      |       |

**Figure 5.9** Split time analysis (ET = elapsed time, ST = split time, %PB = percentage of even-paced personal best time for given 100m section)

paced personal best. For example an athlete with a personal best of two minutes (120s) would be expected to cover each 100m section in 15s. Where this column shows a value of less than 100 per cent, the athlete is running faster than their personal best pace for that 100m section. Where %PB is greater than 100 per cent, the athlete is running slower than their personal best pace for that 100m section. The split times show that athletes 1 and 2 slowed down in the second lap. The elapsed times show that Athlete 1 opened up a 0.4s gap in the first 400m but Athlete 8 closed this to 0.2s by 500m. It also shows that Athlete 8 won the race running slower than his personal best pace in each 100m section.

Other data that can be recorded about middle-distance running performances are the positions of athletes (first, second, third, fourth, etc.) at different points in the race. One disadvantage of using split times or positions is that they sometimes reflect fatigue rather than tactical choice of an athlete. For example, O'Donoghue (2012) analysed 2000m indoor rowing times showing different types of performance. The performances of rowers who did the first half of the race faster than the second half might not always be explained by tactical choice. Some of those athletes might have intended to do a faster second half but were unable to. In events such as the 400m hurdles, touchdown times have been used to analyse performance (Greene *et al.*, 2008). A touchdown time is when an athlete's lead leg touches the ground once a hurdle has been cleared.

The split time data recorded in Figure 5.9 can be displayed in different ways. Brown and O'Donoghue (2006) showed two ways of presenting split time data (Figure 5.10). First, how far an athlete is inside or outside schedule for some target finish time can be evaluated against a fictitious even paced performance. This uses elapsed times rather than split times and has been used effectively in analysing marathon performance where course profile is important (Brown and O'Donoghue, 2006). An alternative way of presenting the data is to determine average speed during each 100m section of a middle-distance race. This is done by dividing the split time for that 100m section into 100m. The higher the value, the faster the athlete is going. Also changes in gradient of the line show where the athlete is speeding up or slowing down. This approach has been useful in analysing sprint running performance using 10m or 20m sections (Bruggerman *et al.*, 1999; Bruggerman and Glad, 1990).

The analysis of timings is also useful in sports such as swimming, cycling and triathlon. The timings may analyse whether a swimmer needs to

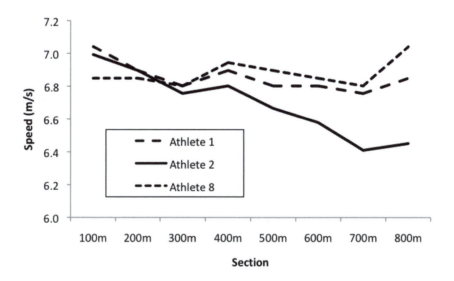

Figure 5.10 A velocity against time chart showing middle distance race performance

concentrate more on their turn or on swimming technique. Cycling times need to be related to course profiles in outdoor road events. In the triathlon, transitions between swimming and cycling or cycling and running can be evaluated to see if an athlete is losing time during these transitions.

## Martial arts

When manual notational analysis has been applied to martial arts, there has been a tendency to report event frequencies (Williams and O'Donoghue, 2006; Hughes and Franks, 2004d: 146–51). Temporal analysis is an important aspect of martial arts that needs greater attention and students are encouraged to evaluate dynamic behaviour within martial arts contests rather than reporting event frequency distributions. The next time you are watching a martial arts contest on television or other media channels, listen to the commentary which is usually by experts with in-depth knowledge of the sport. When the contest is in a given state, the commentators often speculate about the options available to the athletes and which ones have the best opportunity and any risks associated with them. The athletes can then be seen using an option that the commentator has predicted suggesting that there are tactical choices in different situations that have been considered by the athletes prior to those situations occurring. An analysis system can then be developed to record the number of occasions that different outcomes happen when different choices are made in situations of interest to coaches. This can also show transitions between states that occur during a contest. A simple table could be used to show initial state (row) and final state (column) with a tally being recorded for each transition. This approach could also be used to analyse passing patterns for players in a team game.

The analysis of temporal data will be illustrated using a simpler example from martial arts; punch combinations in boxing. Punch combinations are important in boxing and a simple frequency distribution of punch types made cannot provide this information unless commonly occurring combinations are understood. One way of analysing combinations is to record the punches made in a combination within an exploratory notation system. Such a system is used to determine the nature of combinations and which are most popular where no previous information is published. It is not possible to include all possible combinations of punch types within a single tally form because there are so many of them. Imagine that there are nine types of punch and we are looking at combinations of two, three or four punches with only the first four punches of any longer combinations being analysed. This gives 9 × 9 types of combination of two punches, 9 × 9 × 9 types of combination of three punches and 9 × 9 × 9 × 9 types of combination of four punches. This is a total of 7,371 types of combination of two to four punches, most of which will not be observed at all during a contest. Therefore, a more manageable form should be produced to allow combinations and punches performed in isolation to be recorded. Figure 5.11 shows an example of such a sequential system which can be printed on paper or be an Excel spreadsheet where data can be entered directly. Consider the nine punch types used by Harries and O'Donoghue (2012) with their associated one and two letter codes: jabs (J), left (L), right (R), straight (S), uppercut (U), left to the body (LB), right to the body (RB), jab to the body (JB) and straight to the body (SB). Figure 5.11 shows three single punches and two combinations of two punches. The right-most four columns contain the details of punch types performed. If these data are entered into Excel, then the COUNTA function can be used in the seventh

118

| Round | Boxer | Punch 1 | Punch 2 | Punch 3 | Punch 4 |
|-------|-------|---------|---------|---------|---------|
| 1 | Red | J | | | |
| 1 | Blue | J | L | | |
| 1 | Blue | S | | | |
| 1 | Red | J | S | | |
| 1 | Blue | J | | | |
| | | | | | |
| | | | | | |

**Figure 5.11** Partially completed form for boxing combinations and single punches

column to determine the number of punches entered in a row of data. Where one punch has been thrown, it is a single punch. Where two or more punches have been thrown, there is a combination. The '&' operator in Excel is used to combine text strings. Imagine that the first combination 'J' and 'L' are recorded in the cells C3 and D3 with E3 and F3 left blank because there are only two punches in the combination. The eighth column could be programmed '=C3&D3&E3&F3' (in the third row of the spreadsheet) which will combine the text strings giving 'JL'. A simple pivot table can then be used to count the number of each type of single punch and combination that are performed by each boxer.

Where there is published material about commonly performed combinations in boxing, we can simply use a frequency table to record such combinations in a contest of our choice. For example, Harries and O'Donoghue (2012) found that 43 per cent, 58 per cent and 64 per cent of all combinations performed by bantamweight, middleweight and heavyweight boxers respectively were from 12 specific combination types. These are listed in Figure 5.12 which is a frequency table that can be used to tally single punches and other combinations. The data gathering forms shown in Figures 5.11 and 5.12 can be amended to record the outcome of punches by dividing each punch column into two columns. The first of these two columns is used to record the punch type and the second is used to record whether the punch struck the target or not. The data shown in a form such as Figure 5.12 tells us about the tactics of a boxer, what type of single and individual punches they use and which combinations they use most commonly. Where we also have data on punch outcome, we can see how effectively boxers perform different punch types.

| Punch or combination | Red | Blue |
|---|---|---|
| **Single punches** | | |
| Jab | | |
| Left | | |
| Right | | |
| Straight | | |
| Uppercut | | |
| Left to body | | |
| Right to body | | |
| Jab to body | | |
| Straight to body | | |
| | | |
| **Combinations** | | |
| Jab – Straight | | |
| Jab – Jab | | |
| Left – Right | | |
| Right – Left | | |
| Jab – Right | | |
| Left – Straight | | |
| Jab – Left | | |
| Straight – Left | | |
| Uppercut – Left | | |
| Jab – Straight – Jab | | |
| Jab – Uppercut | | |
| Jab – Jab – Straight | | |
| Other | | |

Figure 5.12 Sequential system where we know common combination types

### Technique intensive sports

Analysis of technique is a major area of sports performance in its own right warranting a textbook on its own within the current Sports Performance Analysis series being published by Routledge. Analysis of technique considers how well skills are performed irrespective of whether the tactical choice to perform a skill was appropriate. Lees (2008) classified skills as event skills, major skills and minor skills. Event skills

120

are techniques which constitute the sport, for example jumps and throws in field athletics. Running, swimming and cycling are cyclic sports where the sport is made up almost exclusively of repeated performances of a key skill such as a running stride. Major skills include golf swings and hurdle clearance which are performed repeatedly and have an impact on success in the given sport. Minor skills include different types of kicking the ball in soccer which are important but not as influential to the outcome of a game as major skills. Lees (2008) listed the tennis serve as a minor skill which is debatable. It could be argued to be a major skill in that all points start with a serve and professional players tend to win more points when serving than when receiving.

There are computerised packages such as siliconcoach (siliconcoach, Dunedin, New Zealand) and Dartfish (Dartfish, Fribourg, Switzerland) that allow video frames to be annotated during analysis of technique. These packages also have some quantitative measurement tools for estimating angles and distances of interest. More accurate and detailed analysis of technique is done within the biomechanics discipline using sophisticated equipment and software. The purpose of the current section of this chapter is to consider the role of less ambitious, pen and paper analysis of technique. As mentioned in Chapter 2, technique can be analysed using data collection forms that cross-tabulate body component with temporal phases of the event (Gangstead and Beveridge, 1984). These allow coaches to record notes about event performance. Shorthand notation symbols reduce the volume of writing required during real time observation. Figure 5.13 shows a very general form that can be used by a coach to analyse a skill. Up to six trials of the skill can be analysed. The rows of this general form are completed with important aspects of technique to make the form a more specific form for a given skill. Consider the hammer throw in athletics. How would a student go about turning Figure 5.12 into a specific form for analysing this event? The first thing to do is consult coaching literature about the sport. In the case of the hammer throw, the British Amateur Athletic Board guide written by Carl Johnson (1984) identified areas that that can be included in the form. These are:

(a) The grip

(b) Starting position
   - Foot placement
   - Rear of circle

(c) Swings
- Build-up of hammer momentum
- Rhythm of the throw
- Establishing plane of flight for hammer
- Balance
- Number of swings
- Speed of swings
- Acceleration of the hammer

(d) Entry
- Balance
- Timing
- Relaxation

(e) Turns
- Toe movement
- Angle of swing while turning

(f) Delivery

| Aspect of performance | 1 | 2 | 3 | 4 | 5 | 6 |
|---|---|---|---|---|---|---|
| | | | | | | |
| | | | | | | |
| | | | | | | |
| | | | | | | |
| | | | | | | |
| | | | | | | |
| | | | | | | |
| | | | | | | |
| | | | | | | |
| | | | | | | |
| | | | | | | |
| | | | | | | |
| | | | | | | |
| | | | | | | |

**Figure 5.13** General skill analysis form

122

Other literature (Pedemonte, 1985) discusses other aspects of hammer throwing that can be incorporated in the data collection form. These include projectile mechanics, angle of release, height of release, velocity of release, radius and evolution of turns, rhythm and fluency of turns and swings and the co-ordination between feet and hammer head. The form is typically arranged to follow the phases of the even which is why it has been included under the broad heading of sequential systems.

The hammer-specific version of the form is used by completing a column (1 to 6) for each trial of the skill performed by the athlete. The form is completed for each technical aspect in each trial, leaving the cell blank if there is nothing noteworthy to record. Symbols can be used to record positive aspects ( ✓ ), negative aspects ( ✗ ) and aspects of technique that are too high (↑) or too low (↓). Many variables in sports performance need to be optimal rather than being too high or too low, so both arrow symbols identify areas to be addressed. Unless you are an expert observer of the sport, you will need a video of the skill being performed to carry out the assessment. An expert would typically observe the skill live over a series of trials, building up a mental message to be fed back to the athlete which can be recorded on the form after each trial. Students should repeatedly observe a video recording of the skill being performed and identify aspects requiring attention based on knowledge of the skill and what constitutes a good performance.

## SUMMARY

There are three main types of manual data collection form: scatter diagrams, frequency tables and sequential systems. Sequential systems allow temporal aspects of performance to be record but they do involve further processing of event lists to produce frequency data. Frequency tables require less processing after performances because the frequencies of events are already observable as tallies on the forms. Frequency tables and sequential systems can be used to record the zones of the playing surface where events are performed. However, scatter diagrams are better for recording precise locations of events. The type of form used to record data should be appropriate to the information required about the given aspect of the sport. Systems can use a combination of all three types of form.

# CHAPTER 6

## WORKED EXAMPLES OF MANUAL NOTATION SYSTEMS

### INTRODUCTION

This chapter uses two worked examples to illustrate manual notation systems; one is for tennis and the other is for soccer. The tennis example is a tally system that looks at first and second serves that use slice, flat and kick serve techniques played to the left, middle and right of service boxes when serving to the deuce and advantage courts as well as whether or not the server won the point. If information is needed on any combination of service court, type of serve, serve direction, first or second serve and point outcome by either player in any set, how can the system be developed? Essentially the task is to split data recording areas to factorise the system. Designing it in this way allows queries about any combination of factors to be answered efficiently using data collected with a simple tally system. The second system is a soccer analysis system allowing different types of possession to be evaluated in terms of their outcome. The system is a sequential system that preserves temporal data about the order of possessions. Readers are encouraged to use the system when watching soccer matches to compare their results with classmates' results and discuss sources of disagreement in the data recorded.

### TENNIS EXAMPLE

#### The problem

Figure 6.1 illustrates the observational task in this example. The analyst would typically have an end on view of the court as used when tennis is televised. We wish to analyse the service strategy of each player and how successful they are when making different serve types to different regions of the target service box. We wish to record the following variables about tennis serves:

- Whether the serve was a flat, slice or kick serve.
- Whether the serve was played to the left, middle or right third of the target service court.
- Whether the point was won or lost.

We wish to be able to provide data on:

- Serving to the deuce and advantage courts.
- Points emanating from first and second serves.
- Service strategy in different sets.

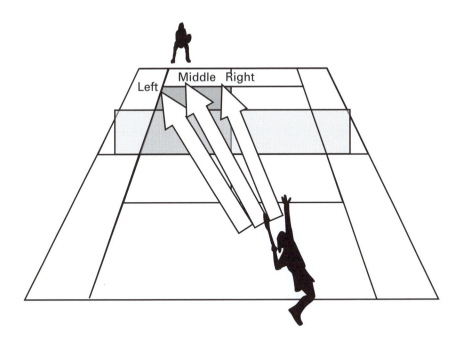

**Figure 6.1** Tennis serve directions

The form is to be used to answer questions about individual variables or variables used in combination. Examples of the type of query that the form needs to help us answer are:

- The number or percentage of points where the first serve is in.
- The number or percentage of points where a flat serve is used.
- The number or percentage of points that are won.

Questions relating to variables used in combination would most often include the percentage of points that are won so that different types of serve can be evaluated in terms of their effectiveness. Examples of the types of such questions include:

- The percentage of points won when the first serve is in.
- The percentage of points won when serving to the deuce court.
- The percentage of points won when using a slice serve.
- The percentage of points won when the first serve is in and was served to the deuce court.
- The percentage of points won when using a flat serve to the advantage court.
- The percentage of points won when using a slice serve on second serve.

There are other queries involving pairs of variables that should be supported, for example:

- The percentage of points where the first serve is in when serving to the deuce court.
- The percentage of points where the first serve is in during the second set.

### Partitioning tallying areas

The requirements for this system do not include the need to look at temporal ordering of points or score lines within games or sets. Therefore, a tally system (or frequency system) is used instead of a sequential system. With two service courts (deuce and advantage), two serves (first and second), three types of serve (flat, slice and kick), three regions of a service court (left, middle and right), we have 2 × 2 × 3 × 3 = 36 combinations of four of the variables where we might wish to look at the percentage of points won within the match or within a given set. There are additional combinations of two or three variables as well as analysing single variables. We need to develop a form that allows any possible combination to be analysed. Consider just two of the variables: whether the first serve was in or a second serve was required and whether the counting serve was played to the deuce or advantage court.

When designing the form, we need to consider that it could be used to derive the information required for the previously listed queries. The most challenging aspect of this is to answer questions about combined variables. To give an idea of how to do this and how not to do it, we will consider the example on a smaller scale using just two variables; whether the first serve was in or not and whether the point was won or not. Figure 6.2 can be used answer questions about these variables in isolation, but it fails to answer questions about the two variables in combination. A total of 30 points has been played and we can see that the first serve was in on 17/30 points (56.7 per cent) and that the server won the point on 20/30 points (66.7 per cent). However, we cannot tell the percentage of points won when the first serve was in or when a second serve was required. Another disadvantage of Figure 6.2 is that we need to tally each point twice; once to show whether the point was from a first or second serve and once to indicate the outcome of the point. Imagine if we added all of the other variables as well. There would be six different frequencies the serve would have to be added to: the serve, the service court, the serve type, the region of the service court, the outcome of the point and the set being played.

To be able to answer questions about the two variables in combination, we need to 'factorise' the form. We need to partition the tallying area for

| Variable | Value | Tally |
|----------|-------|-------|
| Service | 1st | ⊞⊞ ⊞⊞ ⊞⊞ II |
| | 2nd | ⊞⊞ ⊞⊞ III |
| Outcome | Win | ⊞⊞ ⊞⊞ ⊞⊞ ⊞⊞ |
| | Lose | ⊞⊞ ⊞⊞ |

Figure 6.2 A poor attempt that fails to analyse variables in combination

first serve points and the area for second serve points to record and show different tallies for points won and lost in each case. This might look like Figure 6.3. Here we can still see that 20 points have been won overall and 10 points have been lost. This is done by adding the values for first and second serves. We can also still see that the first serve was in on 17 points and a second serve was required on 13 points. This is done by adding totals for points won and lost. Because Figure 6.3 has partitioned areas relating to first and second serve based on point outcome, we can also answer questions about the variables in combination. There were 11/17 points won when the first serve was in (64.7 per cent) and 9/13 points won when a second serve was required (69.2 per cent). Perhaps this player should play the first serve deliberately out because they win a greater percentage of points when using a second serve! Another advantage of Figure 6.3 is that each point only has to be tallied once rather than twice. This is because each of the four tallying cells is related to a service (row) and outcome (column). Now try to apply partitioning when designing the form for all of the variables of interest.

## A solution

Figure 6.4 is the author's solution to this exercise. The idea was to start with a single area to record the points and then split this into two rows; one for points where the first serve was in and one for points where a second serve is required. Each of these rows is then split in two; one partition for serves to the deuce court and one partition for serves to the advantage court. This gives four tallying areas in a 2 × 2 table at this stage. We can then split each column into three to represent the left, middle and right thirds of the service courts. We will now have 12 cells in our data collection form. Each row is split into three rows to record the three different types of serve (flat, slice and kick). Finally, we split each of the rows

| | | Outcome | |
|---|---|---|---|
| | | Win | Lose |
| Service | 1st | ⊞⊞ ⊞⊞ I | ⊞⊞ I |
| | 2nd | ⊞⊞ IIII | IIII |

Figure 6.3 An improved form allowing combinations of variables

| Serve | Serve type | Outcome | Deuce | | | Advantage | | |
|---|---|---|---|---|---|---|---|---|
| | | | Left | Middle | Right | Left | Middle | Right |
| 1st | Flat | Win | | | | | | |
| | | Lose | | | | | | |
| | Slice | Win | | | | | | |
| | | Lose | | | | | | |
| | Kick | Win | | | | | | |
| | | Lose | | | | | | |
| 2nd | Flat | Win | | | | | | |
| | | Lose | | | | | | |
| | Slice | Win | | | | | | |
| | | Lose | | | | | | |
| | Kick | Win | | | | | | |
| | | Lose | | | | | | |

Figure 6.4 A solution for five of the variables. Each set would be analysed on a separate form

in the form into two rows to record points won and lost. This results in 72 tallying area within a 2 × 2 × 3 × 3 × 2 structure. One thing that has not been done in Figure 6.4 is dealing with sets. Once the form gets partitioned to this extent, it is recommended that separate forms are used for each set. This will allow separate sets to be analysed and totals determined from the forms for the different sets to obtain overall match statistics.

This is a solution rather than the only possible solution. The decision about which variables should be rows or columns may be different in readers' solutions. The author decided to make service court and left, middle and right thirds of the service courts columns because he often analyses tennis while watching television coverage. Television coverage of tennis typically shows points viewing from behind one of the baselines. The form works well when the player is serving from the near baseline (as in Figure 6.1) but may need to be turned around when the player is serving from the far baseline.

One possibility is to turn the form upside down when this happens and duplicate the headings upside down at the bottom and right of the form. This is shown in Figure 6.5. In general, the most used variables should

Serving from near end

| Serve | Type | Outc | Deuce | | | Advantage | | | | | |
|---|---|---|---|---|---|---|---|---|---|---|---|
| | | | Left | Mid | Right | Left | Mid | Right | | | |
| 1st | Flat | Win | | | | | | | uiW | | |
| | | Lose | | | | | | | əsoꞀ | ʇɐlℲ | |
| | Slice | Win | | | | | | | uiW | | |
| | | Lose | | | | | | | əsoꞀ | əɔilS | |
| | Kick | Win | | | | | | | uiW | | |
| | | Lose | | | | | | | əsoꞀ | ʞɔiʞ | ʇsꞁ |
| 2nd | Flat | Win | | | | | | | uiW | | |
| | | Lose | | | | | | | əsoꞀ | ʇɐlℲ | |
| | Slice | Win | | | | | | | uiW | | |
| | | Lose | | | | | | | əsoꞀ | əɔilS | |
| | Kick | Win | | | | | | | uiW | | |
| | | Lose | | | | | | | əsoꞀ | ʞɔiʞ | puᄅ |
| | | | ʇɟəꞀ | piW | ʇɥɓiꞍ | ʇɟəꞀ | piW | ʇɥɓiꞍ | | | |
| | | | | əɔuəᗡ | | | əɓɐʇuɐʌp∀ | | ɔʇuO | ədʎꞀ | əʌɹəS |

Serving from far end

Figure 6.5 The form is modified so as it can be used upside down when the player serves from the far side of the court

be designed into the form first. For example, overall service rates from first and second serve points are widely used in tennis research and media coverage. Service court (deuce or advantage) was considered the next most important variable according to how this author would use the form. Having the 36 tallying areas for first serve points located together makes it easier for users to determine totals for such points. Determining statistics for service type (such as the kick serve) is a little harder because the 24 tallying areas are located more remotely.

## Exercises

Let us consider the completed version of the form shown in Figure 6.6. From the data recorded in the form, determine the following:

■ The percentage of points where the first serve was in.
■ The percentage of points won when the first serve was in.
■ The percentage of points won when a second serve was required.
■ The percentage of points won when serving to the deuce court.

130

- The percentage of points won when serving to the deuce court and the first serve was in.
- The percentage of points won when a flat serve was used.
- The percentage of points won when the slice serve was used to the advantage court when a second serve was required.
- The percentage of first serve points that were served to the middle third of the service box (combining deuce and advantage courts).
- The percentage of second serve points that were served to the middle third of the service box (combining deuce and advantage courts).
- The percentage of all points where flat, slice and kick serves were used.
- The percentage of first serve points where flat, slice and kick serves were used.
- The percentage of second serve points where flat, slice and kick serves were used.
- The percentage of points won when serving to the right third of the deuce court, where a flat serve was used and the first serve was in.

**Serving from near end**

| Serve | Type | Outc | Deuce | | | Advantage | | |
|-------|------|------|-------|-----|-------|-----------|-----|-------|
| | | | Left | Mid | Right | Left | Mid | Right |
| 1st | Flat | Win | III | I | II | IIII | | II |
| | | Lose | I | | I | I | I | |
| | Slice | Win | I | I | I | III | I | |
| | | Lose | I | | | II | | |
| | Kick | Win | | | | | | II |
| | | Lose | I | | | | | I |
| 2nd | Flat | Win | | I | | I | II | |
| | | Lose | | II | | | I | |
| | Slice | Win | I | II | | | I | |
| | | Lose | I | I | | | III | |
| | Kick | Win | | | I | | I | I |
| | | Lose | | I | | | | |

(The right-hand portion of the form repeats the same layout inverted for "Serving from far end", with columns Serve / Type / Outc, Win/Lose for Flat, Slice, Kick serves for 1st and 2nd, and Deuce / Advantage courts with Left, Mid, Right.)

Figure 6.6 A completed version of the tennis data collection form

**worked examples of manual systems**

## Solutions to exercises

- The percentage of points where the first serve was in. **30/50 = 60 per cent**
- The percentage of points won when the first serve was in. **21/30 = 70 per cent**
- The percentage of points won when a second serve was required. **11/20 = 55 per cent**
- The percentage of points won when serving to the deuce court. **14/23 = 60.9 per cent**
- The percentage of points won when serving to the deuce court and the first serve was in. **9/13 = 69.2 per cent**
- The percentage of points won when a flat serve was used. **16/23 = 69.6 per cent**
- The percentage of points won when the slice serve was used to the advantage court when a second serve was required. **1/4 = 25 per cent note we needed 6 cells for this but only two are populated**
- The percentage of first serve points that were served to the middle third of the service box. (combining deuce and advantage courts). **4/30 = 13.3 per cent**
- The percentage of second serve points that were served to the middle third of the service box? (combining deuce and advantage courts). **15/20 = 75 per cent**
- The percentage of all points where flat, slice and kick serves were used. **Flat 23/50 = 46 per cent, Slice 19/50 = 38 per cent, Kick 8/50 = 16 per cent**
- The percentage of first serve points where flat, slice and kick serves were used. **Flat 16/30 = 53.3 per cent, Slice 10/30 = 33.3 per cent, Kick 4/30 = 13.3 per cent**
- The percentage of second serve points where flat, slice and kick serves were used. **Flat 7/20 = 35 per cent, Slice 9/20 = 45 per cent, Kick 4/20 = 20 per cent**
- The percentage of points won when serving to the right third of the deuce court, where a flat serve was used and the first serve was in. **2/3 = 66.7 per cent**

132

## Analysis of data

The data may need to be analysed immediately after a match to produce information. This might involve calculating percentages using a calculator on a mobile phone. It is best to write row and column totals in the margins on the form to avoid counting the same tallies on multiple occasions. The analyst could also have calculated the most commonly used statistics prior to meeting with the coach to give a head start to the feedback which would only be held up by the need for any unanticipated queries. This is a lot easier if two copies of the form are used (one for each player) than if ten copies are used (one for each player in each of five sets played). This is because all of the data for a given player is on a single form when individual sets do not need to be analysed.

If the analyst has more time, the 72 frequencies tallied in the cells of each form can be keyed into a pre-programmed Microsoft Excel spreadsheet which determines the frequency and percentage of points played as well as the percentage points won for different conditions and different combinations of conditions.

## Temporal analysis

The system shown in Figure 6.6 cannot record temporal data which might be important to understand. For example, some forthcoming opponents may have a serving strategy that includes temporal patterns. Some players might serve more to the right of the advantage court if the previous point to the deuce court was to the middle than if it was to the left or right of the deuce court. Figure 6.6 only shows the totals at the end of the match without any such temporal information. Figure 6.7 is an example of a system that might be used for temporal analysis of serving strategy. The outcome of the point is not important as we are analysing serving strategy irrespective of the effectiveness of the serve. A further point about the data collection form in Figure 6.7 is that it is only used with first serves irrespective of whether they are played in or are faults. There are two parts of the form; one for serves to the deuce court and one for serves to the advantage court. The rows represent the previous service point (which will usually be to the other service court) while the columns represent the current point. Therefore, details of the first point are not entered because there was no previous point. The form allows us

| Previous point (advantage court) | | Current point (advantage court) | | | | | | | | |
|---|---|---|---|---|---|---|---|---|---|---|
| | | Flat | | | Slice | | | Kick | | |
| | | L | M | R | L | M | R | L | M | R |
| Flat | L | | | | | | | | | |
| | M | | | | | | | | | |
| | R | | | | | | | | | |
| Slice | L | | | | | | | | | |
| | M | | | | | | | | | |
| | R | | | | | | | | | |
| Kick | L | | | | | | | | | |
| | M | | | | | | | | | |
| | R | | | | | | | | | |

| Previous point (deuce court) | | Current point (deuce court) | | | | | | | | |
|---|---|---|---|---|---|---|---|---|---|---|
| | | Flat | | | Slice | | | Kick | | |
| | | L | M | R | L | M | R | L | M | R |
| Flat | L | | | | | | | | | |
| | M | | | | | | | | | |
| | R | | | | | | | | | |
| Slice | L | | | | | | | | | |
| | M | | | | | | | | | |
| | R | | | | | | | | | |
| Kick | L | | | | | | | | | |
| | M | | | | | | | | | |
| | R | | | | | | | | | |

Figure 6.7 A possible hand notation form to analyse temporal aspects of service strategy

to tally the number of times each of the nine strategies (3 serve types × 3 directions) is used for each of the nine strategies used in the previous point.

The usefulness of this system is questionable because even in a quite long five-set match, there may only be about 150 service points for the player; 80 to the deuce court and 70 to the advantage court because some games are completed when serving to the deuce court. This means that many of the 162 cells in the form will not have any data recorded and other cells may have one or two serves recorded. However, data for serve types on their own (or serve directions on their own) could be considered to allow more representative data to be analysed. Another issue with the usefulness of the form is that the first serve of a game is different from other serves played to the deuce court. This is because the previous service point was two games earlier. Another issue is whether we include service points played within tie-breakers during the analysis. A further issue is that the temporal data is restricted to pairs of points rather than sequences of three or four points.

A more serious issue with the form in Figure 6.7 is its usability. Imagine the player serves a flat serve to the right of the deuce court in the first point (which is not recorded because there is no previous point). The user needs to place their finger on the 'Flat'-'R' row of the half of the form to be used for the next point. This is the third row of the form and represents what happened in the previous point as we observe the second point. The second point sees a kick serve played to the middle of the advantage court. The user, therefore, adds to the tally in row 3 column 8 for serves to the advantage court. This represents that the kick serve to the middle (column 8) has been used when the previous point was a flat serve to the right (row 3). Having recorded this second point, the user must now place their finger on row 8 ('Kick'-'M') of the section of the form used to record serves to the deuce court. This is because the third point is served to the deuce court and the previous point was a kick serve to the middle of the advantage court. This process continues and requires considerable concentration, especially if we have to remember the last point of one service game until the player's next service game. This system is so awkward, it would be better using a sequential system which could be analysed later to tally frequencies for different strategies used in pairs of service points. In Chapters 7 and 8, when reading about computerised systems, users should think about this particular system and how much easier it is to enter and analyse data in a computerised version of the system.

## SOCCER POSSESSION EXAMPLE

### The problem

We are interested in possessions and capitalising on possessions in soccer matches. Each possession is characterised by the team in possession of the ball, the way the possession started, the area of the playing surface where the possession started and whether the possession resulted in a scoring opportunity or not. The end of the possession is either a score or a change of possession to the other team. Therefore, we do not need to record the details about the end of possessions because they can be seen by examining the next possession to occur in the match. For example, if one team loses the ball with a pass that was intercepted by the opponents, then the opponents' next possession commences with an interception.

A possession may include more than one shot; for example a team may take a shot which hits the bar, regain the ball after the rebound and take another shot before the possession ends. Therefore, we need to consider how we record shots and how we analyse these. Are we interested in the percentage of different types of possession that lead to scoring opportunities? Are we interested in the number of shots that result from different types of possession? We will develop the system so that both types of information can be provided.

There are two teams ('Us' and 'Them'). There are nine areas of the pitch as shown in Figure 6.8. 'L', 'C' and 'R' are used to represent the left, central and right hand channels of the pitch respectively, while 'D', 'M' and 'A' are used to represent the defending, middle and attacking thirds with respect to the team. Users of the system need to familiarise themselves with these letters and make sure they do not confuse 'C' and 'M' which could easily have been used the other way round when designing the system. The other thing we need to consider is whether we use the areas with respect to our own team; in other words 'DL' is the left wing of our defending third and the right wing of their attacking third. The alternative is to express location with respect to each team's direction of play; in other words 'DL' is always used to represent the left wing of the defending third for the team in possession of the ball. We will use this second way because it allows direct comparison between the teams.

Possessions alternate between the two teams. The methods of starting a possession are listed below:

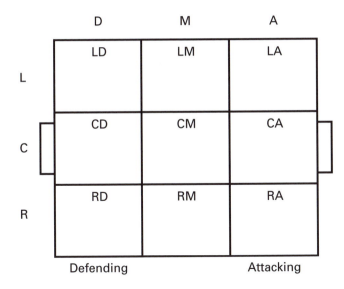

**Figure 6.8** Locations of the pitch

- Kick off (at the beginning of a match period or after conceding a goal).
- Successful tackle.
- Interception including saves by the goalkeeper.
- Throw in where the ball has been played off the side of the pitch by the opponents.
- Corner where the opponents have played to ball over their own back line.
- Goal kick where the opponents have played the ball over the back line (pass or shot).
- Free kick where the team that had been in possession has committed an offence meaning the other team gets a free kick; for example hand ball or off side.

## A sequential system

Possessions alternate between the two teams. We could use two-letter codes to record possession types:

# 137

- KO: Kick off.
- TK: Successful tackle.
- IN: Interception.
- TI: Throw in.
- CO: Corner.
- GK: Goal kick.
- FK: Free kick.

These two-letter codes are just one way of recording events as shorthand symbols could be used instead, especially if it is easier to write them. The end of one possession is signified by a new possession for the opposing team. The only other way that a possession can end is where the particular match period ends.

There are some issues that analysts need to consider when using this system. First, what constitutes a possession? If one of our players passes the ball and an opponent manages to touch the ball without controlling it and the ball travels on to be received by one of our own players, did we temporarily lose possession of the ball? Technically we did lose the ball, but we might not want to analyse possessions where a team was never in control of the ball. A second issue is that we are not recording all free kicks, we are only recording those that result in a possession change. So if our team has the ball and an opponent commits a foul and we are awarded a free kick, we do not record it because it is still our possession. This has implications for the way in which the information is used. We might see a high conversion rate of goals scored for possessions commencing with a tackle or interception. This may be interpreted as the team being good at capitalising on possessions where they need to quickly make the transition from defending to attacking. However, some of these possessions might have been interrupted by free kicks being awarded. In situations where this happens and goals are scored, the team and their opponents were able to set up their formations before the restart and the outcome of the possession does not really reflect the ability to make the transition from defence to attack during open play. If coaches start to make these kinds of interpretations of the data, the analyst should be honest with the coaches and warn that there are free kicks in the middle of some possessions. A future version of the system might have to be developed where a possession outcome is 'Retained' and is used to signify that the possession ended but the same team will be in possession of the ball when the subsequent free kick is taken. Similarly,

138

there may be throw ins and corners that are not recorded if a team plays the ball off an opponent and it goes out of play for the throw in or corner. This might be problematic for the coach who might be interested in conversion rates from all corner kicks and throw ins. If one thinks of soccer, a minority of corner kicks happen because a team in control of the ball plays the ball out behind its own back line. However, if we insist on possession being a state that alternates between the teams and a possession only counts where a team has control of the ball for at least one touch of the ball then some throw ins and corner kicks will not be recorded.

Figure 6.9 shows a sequential system that could be used to capture the data. Our team kicks off at 0 mins 0s in the centre of the pitch. The opponents intercept the ball in the centre of their defensive third (centre of our attacking third) after 15s. Seven seconds later, we regain the ball making a successful tackle on the right wing of the central third of the pitch. What has happened is that having made the tackle, the ball was moved to the centre of the attacking third and a shot taken which the opposition saved. We have not actually recorded that the keeper made a save. The way the possession change was recorded, the shot could have struck the post before being received by an opposing defender or the shot could have been blocked by an opposition defender before the opponents took control of the ball. On 34s, the opponents take the ball (the keeper saved it and we recorded this as an interception by them in the centre of their defensive third), moving the ball to the other end of the pitch and score against us. We restart the match with a kick off in the middle of the pitch after 48s.

| Time | Team | Possession | Area | Outcome |
|------|------|------------|------|---------|
| 00:00 | Us | KO | CM | |
| 00:15 | Them | IN | CD | |
| 00:22 | Us | TK | RM | Shot |
| 00:34 | Them | IN | CD | Score |
| 00:48 | Us | KO | CM | |
| | | | | |
| | | | | |

Figure 6.9 Sequential system to record possessions in soccer

Once the sequential system has been used to record the possessions within the match, this list of possessions can be analysed to determine different types of output including:

- A summary table or column chart showing the volume of possessions starting in different ways and the proportion of these resulting in shots or goals. This can be done for each team individually.
- Similar summary tables or charts showing the volume of possessions starting in different areas of the playing surface and the proportion of these resulting in shots or goals.
- A cross-tabulation of possession type against following possession type allowing the full breakdown of possession changes to be displayed for each possession type.

Imagine a situation where a possession led to more than one shot; for example hitting the post and then scoring a goal from another shot after the ball rebounded off the post. We would record 'Shot, Goal' in the outcome of this particular possession. When counting the number of possessions of the given type or starting area that result in shots being taken or goals being scored, we would only record that this possession led to a goal. The additional shot would not be included in the calculation of the percentage of such possessions that lead to goals or scoring opportunities. If, however, we did wish to know the number of shots coming from particular possession types, we would include this additional shot in the calculation.

Having to write down 'Them', 'IN', 'CD' (for example) requires the analyst to look at what they are writing rather than the match. While they are writing, they might miss another possession change, meaning the system is difficult to use live. The system might be satisfactory for post-match analysis of a match video which can be paused on each possession change, but live notation is difficult. The operator might make mistakes coding locations. Figure 6.10 is a version of the system that simply requires the analyst to tick the team, possession type, area where the possession commenced and outcome. This requires less time for writing and allows the analyst to spend a greater amount of time actually observing the match. There is still a need to record the time of possession changes. However, this may not be necessary for all possessions. The analyst might choose to periodically record times for possession changes after stoppages in play. This version of the system has more of a chance

140

| Time | Team | | Possession | | | | | | | Area | | | Outcome | |
|---|---|---|---|---|---|---|---|---|---|---|---|---|---|---|
| | U | T | KO | TK | IN | TI | CO | GK | FK | D | M | A | shot | Score |
| 00:00 | ✓ | | ✓ | | | | | | | | ✓ | | | |
| 00:15 | | ✓ | | | ✓ | | | | | ✓ | | | | |
| 00:22 | ✓ | | | ✓ | | | | | | | ✓ | | ✓ | |
| 00:34 | | ✓ | | | ✓ | | | | | ✓ | | | | ✓ |
| 00:48 | ✓ | | ✓ | | | | | | | | ✓ | | | |
| 01:35 | | ✓ | | | ✓ | | | | | ✓ | | | | |

Figure 6.10 An improved version of the soccer possession analysis system

of being used live than the version in Figure 6.9. However, this is still a challenging task and system users would need to undergo sufficient training to be able to use the system live.

The system has advantages and disadvantages over a tallying system. The advantage is that temporal information is recorded allowing periods of territorial domination to be seen where one team cannot get into the other's defending third for a long period of time. This does assume, however, that the location where a possession ended was the most advanced location during the possession. In reality, it is possible that a team might have entered the attacking third, passed the ball back into the middle third and lost possession in the middle third. Only the locations of possession changes are recorded meaning that this last third entry will be missed by the recording process. The system allows the series of possessions prior to shots and scores to be analysed. The disadvantage of the systems shown in Figures 6.9 and 6.10 is that the chronological list of possessions needs further processing to provide summary information. A tally system displays frequencies for different combinations of possession types, areas where they start and outcomes that can transformed into percentages more easily. A further disadvantage of the system shown in Figure 6.10 is that it uses more paper than the system shown in Figure 6.9.

## Summary analysis form

Given that the data need further analysis, we need an additional form to the data collection form shown in Figure 6.10. Figure 6.11 shows a summary form that can be used to record the frequency of each possession type in each area of the pitch as well as the frequency of those possessions where shots were taken or scores occurred. These frequencies are determined by counting up the possessions entered into the data collection form (Figure 6.10). Overall totals for each possession type and each pitch area should also be determined from this information. Totals for broader pitch areas such as the three-thirds of the pitch (defensive, middle or attacking) or the three channels (left, centre or right) should also be produced. If we are not interested in temporal aspects of performance, Figure 6.11 is close to the type of tallying system that could be used to collect the data in the first place.

## Exercise

Use the forms shown in Figures 6.10 and 6.11 to analyse possession changes in soccer. Modify the system to allow restarts where possession does not change, for example corners, throw ins and free kicks where the team previously in possession of the ball has retained possession for these restarts. As an example of the type of play that is represented differently between your system and Figure 6.10, consider the period between 48s into the match and 1 min 35s into the match shown in Figure 6.10. At 00:48, we kick off after conceding a goal. During the possession, we

# 142

| Channel | Possession | Defending 3rd | | | Middle 3rd | | | Attacking 3rd | | | Total | | |
|---|---|---|---|---|---|---|---|---|---|---|---|---|---|
| | | Freq | shot | score | Freq | shot | score | Freq | shot | score | Freq | shot | score |
| Left | KO | | | | | | | | | | | | |
| | TK | | | | | | | | | | | | |
| | IN | | | | | | | | | | | | |
| | TI | | | | | | | | | | | | |
| | CO | | | | | | | | | | | | |
| | GK | | | | | | | | | | | | |
| | FK | | | | | | | | | | | | |
| Centre | KO | | | | 2 | | | | | | 2 | | |
| | TK | | | | | | | | | | | | |
| | IN | | | | | | | | | | | | |
| | TI | | | | | | | | | | | | |
| | CO | | | | | | | | | | | | |
| | GK | | | | | | | | | | | | |
| | FK | | | | | | | | | | | | |
| Right | KO | | | | | | | | | | | | |
| | TK | | | | 1 | 1 | | | | | 1 | 1 | |
| | IN | | | | | | | | | | | | |
| | TI | | | | | | | | | | | | |
| | CO | | | | | | | | | | | | |
| | GK | | | | | | | | | | | | |
| | FK | | | | | | | | | | | | |
| All | KO | | | | 2 | | | | | | 2 | | |
| | TK | | | | 1 | 1 | | | | | 1 | 1 | |
| | IN | | | | | | | | | | | | |
| | TI | | | | | | | | | | | | |
| | CO | | | | | | | | | | | | |
| | GK | | | | | | | | | | | | |
| | FK | | | | | | | | | | | | |

**Figure 6.11** Summary analysis form showing outcomes of different possession types starting in different areas of the pitch. The values shown are for 'us' derived from Figure 6.9 or Figure 6.10

make a long pass towards the penalty area, but an opposition defender deflects the ball out of play so it does not reach the penalty area immediately. We have a corner, but because it is still our possession the corner is not recorded in Figure 6.10. The corner is taken at 01:30 and an opposing defender clears the ball with a header (recorded as an interception) starting a new possession for the opposition at 01:35. The header was made in the centre of the opposition defensive third and so this is where the new possession is deemed to have started.

**A solution**

Figure 6.12 shows a solution that allows consecutive possessions for the same team to be recorded where possession is retained. Note the

| Time | Team | | Possession | | | | | | | Area | | | Outcome | | |
|---|---|---|---|---|---|---|---|---|---|---|---|---|---|---|---|
| | U | T | KO | TK | IN | TI | CO | GK | FK | D | M | A | Retained | shot | Score |
| 00:00 | | ✓ | ✓ | | | | | | | | ✓ | | | | |
| 00:15 | | ✓ | | | ✓ | | | | | ✓ | | | | | |
| 00:22 | ✓ | | | ✓ | | | | | | | ✓ | | ✓ | | |
| 00:34 | | ✓ | | | ✓ | | | | | ✓ | | | | ✓ | |
| 00:48 | ✓ | | ✓ | | | | | | | | ✓ | | | | |
| 01:35 | | ✓ | | | ✓ | | | | | ✓ | | | | | |

Figure 6.12 An improved version of the system

144

additional row of data at 01:30 and the additional outcome class (Retained) that were not included in Figure 6.10. Our team's possession that commenced with the kick off at 00:48 is now split into two possessions. The first of these possessions commenced at 00:48 and ended with the ball being retained by our team. The second of these possessions commended at 01:30 when our team took a corner. This is just one solution and some readers may view the 'retained' column of the Outcome area as being redundant because we can see if the team retained possession in the next row of the form anyway. This redundant information has been included in this version because it eases the analysis to be done later. The summary analysis form shown in Figure 6.11 would need to change so that the sets of three columns ('Freq', 'shot', 'score') included a fourth column where possession is retained.

## SUMMARY

This chapter has built on Chapter 5 by describing two systems: a tally system and a sequential system. The tally system used for analysing service strategy in tennis is capable of providing reasonably quick feedback of overall performance statistics from a tennis match. However, tally systems are not good for analysing temporal aspects. The sequential system used for analysing soccer possessions does allow analysis of temporal aspects of performance. However, the main disadvantage of sequential systems is that further analysis of the data is necessary to provide match statistics for coaches.

# CHAPTER 7

## GUIDELINES FOR COMPUTERISED PERFORMANCE ANALYSIS SYSTEMS

### INTRODUCTION

This chapter covers the use of computerised systems for sports performance analysis. There are general purpose video analysis packages that can be tailored for analysis of performances in sports of the user's choice. These packages allow the event types that occur within a sport to be defined, effectively creating a sport specific system using the package. Some software systems are special purpose and have been created for specific sports. These include commercially available packages for popular sports as well as systems specifically developed and used within particular coaching set ups or scientific research projects. There are other packages that do not involve video analysis but which can be used for quantitative analysis of sports performances.

sportscode is used as an example of a general purpose match analysis package. In designing a Code Window to capture event data, the analyst must be aware of the potential use of Matrices (of events by value labels) to provide outputs of interest to coaches and players. The different types of events (fixed duration and variable duration) are covered as well as value labels that are used as modifiers of events. Activation and exclusive links between events are described and guidance for their use is given. The process of tagging a match video and analysing the resulting Matrices are discussed. The chapter also covers interactive video feedback and the creation of highlight movies. Some mention is given of other packages, such as Focus X2, Nacsports and Dartfish, due to their different ways of representing and analysing behaviour.

The features of special purpose commercial packages used with soccer and cricket are described and two special purpose systems developed for use in rugby union and tennis research are also covered. The relative advantages and disadvantages of general purpose and special purpose packages are listed.

There are three types of manual notation system: sequential systems, frequency tables and scatter diagrams. We do not need to make a decision between using a frequency table or a sequential system when developing computerised systems. This is because the computer can rapidly process sequential data producing summary frequency tables. This is flexible and can be done for any combination of variables required. Scatter diagrams can also be used to enter event locations into a computerised system. These can then be stored with other event data such as player, team, event type, time and outcome.

## GENERAL PURPOSE VIDEO TAGGING PACKAGES

### Representation of behaviour and data entry

Figure 7.1 shows the different ways that two different packages represent behaviour in sport; Focus X2 and sportscode. A match can be abstracted to be a series of events. Some packages, such as Focus X2 (Elite Sports Analysis, Delgaty Bay, Fife Scotland), represent an event as being performed at an instant in time. For example, a pass in soccer could be tagged at the point in time when a player's foot struck the ball. The user defines a pre-roll period and a post-roll period to be used if the event is to be shown as a video clip. The pre-roll is the period before the event and the post-roll is the period after the event. These could be 3s and 5s respectively allowing the viewers to see 3s of play leading up to the pass and the 5s afterwards allowing outcome of the pass to be observed. The amount of pre-roll and post-roll can vary between different event types. It is also possible in Focus X2 to allow the video to play on from the time of the event until the viewer pauses the video rather than defining a specific post-roll. This is useful where the amount of video we wish to view varies within event type. For example, in badminton we could have an event 'point' which starts as soon as a player serves. Not all points are the same duration and so we would not wish to impose a uniform post-roll period on all points. This works well when video sequences are being shown interactively using the package during debriefing sessions. However, if we wish to save highlights into a summary video, it is necessary to define a post-roll period which might not be suitable for all points meaning some additional video editing will be necessary or different post-rolls will have to be set up for individual points. Alternatively, each instance of a rally needs to have an individual post-roll period defined.

Having behaviour abstracted to a series of discrete events of no duration means any behaviours of non-zero duration need to be represented by instantaneous start and end events. Examples of such behaviours occur in coach behaviour, running events and time-motion analysis. Event Lists can be processed to allow durations between event times (representing the start of behaviours or movements) to be determined by subtraction.

sportscode (Sportstec Inc, Warriewood, New South Wales, Australia) differs from Focus X2 in that it uses a timeline. The timeline is a graphical representation of behaviours that have been tagged which can be exported as an Event List for processing if needed. The events in sportscode typically have duration with different start and end times for event instances. The user can tag the start and end of such an event. Alternatively the end of an event can be marked at the point some other event commences (if the two event types are exclusively linked). Where event types are exclusively linked, only one of them is allowed at any point in the timeline. Other event types can have the same duration for all instances meaning that the user only has to tag them once and predefined lead and lag times are used to mark the start and end of each instance on the timeline. It is technically possible to have some instantaneous events in sportscode where lead time and lag time are set to zero seconds. This would, however, only display a single frame for the event but could be useful for marking events that are not to be shown as video clips. Figure 7.1 shows how events could be represented on a sportscode timeline when lag times are set and when they are not set.

Events can have other information about them recorded in both Focus X2 and sportscode. For example, when a pass is made in soccer, we may wish to know the team and player making the pass, the area of the pitch where the pass was played and the outcome of the pass. In Focus X2, a Category Set is defined to represent the behaviours of interest within the given sport. A Category Set is composed of categories such as event type, team, player, pitch area and outcome as shown in Figure 7.2. When an event is entered, a value is needed for each of the categories. The event

148

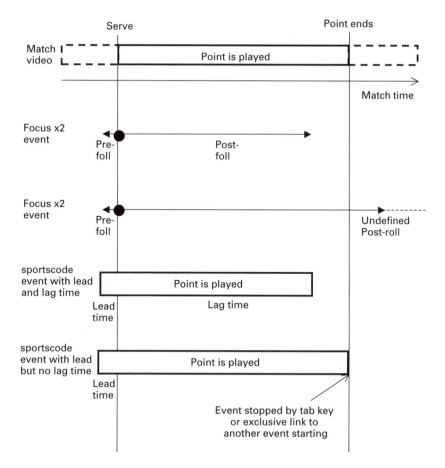

**Figure 7.1** Abstraction of behaviour in Focus X2 and sportscode

is timed on one category and logged on another. For example, the system could be set up so that events are timed when a value is entered for the event type category. This preserves the video time of the event while the user enters values for the other categories. Where a video is being coded live as it is being captured onto computer disk, the user cannot pause the video to enter values for the other categories. So preserving the time of the event as being the time at which the event type was entered ensures the event is tagged at the correct time irrespective of how long the user takes to enter the other values. The system could be set up to log the event

| Category | Values | | | | | |
|---|---|---|---|---|---|---|
| Event type (timed) | Pass | Shot | Tackle | Keeping | Restart | Interception |
| Team | Us | | | Opposition | | |
| Player | 1 | 2 | 3 | 4 | 5 | 6 | 7 | 8 | 9 | 10 | 11 |
| Pitch area | DL | DC | DR | ML | MC | MR | AL | AC | AR |
| Outcome (logged) | Successful | | | Unsuccessful | | |

**Figure 7.2** A category set in Focus X2

(completing it in the Event List) when a value is entered for the outcome category. In between entering a value for the event type category and the outcome category, the user should enter values for the remaining categories. Some categories can be set up to have 'sticky buttons' so that the previously used value for that category is used by default. For example, in tennis, the player serving will be the same as the player serving the previous point unless there is a change of games or an odd number of points has been played within a tiebreaker.

There may be some behaviours in sport, where some information is needed for some event types but not for others. For example, in tennis we may have a category 'point type' with seven values: ace, double fault, serve winner, return winner, server to net first, receiver to net first or baseline rally (O'Donoghue and Ingram, 2001). If a point is an ace, double fault, serve winner or return winner then we do not need to enter a value for whether a point finishes on a winner or error. This is an example of a variant record where the data structure for an event differs depending on the event type. In Focus X2, a value needs to be entered for every category. Therefore, it may be necessary to have some 'N/A' (not applicable) values for some categories.

In sportscode, the system is defined using a Code Window that contains two types of button: event buttons and labels. Event buttons are used to represent observable behaviours that are to be recorded in the timeline. As has already been mentioned, some of these event types have pre-defined durations. Other event types have varying durations. A set of event buttons can be exclusively linked meaning that when any one of them is activated, any existing active event within the set of events is deactivated as the new event commences. Some events are allowed to occur in parallel. For example, a broad possession event in soccer can be active at the same time as individual behaviour events such as passes and shots that occur during possessions. Activation links can be used for events to trigger other events. For example, in soccer we may have events representing short passes and long passes with both of these event types activating a more general pass event that is recorded in parallel. Label buttons are used to store other information within events. For example, the team, player, area of the pitch and outcome can all be labels used to add details to event records. Because we can enter as many or as few label buttons as are needed to modify an active event, variant records are possible in sportscode and we do not need to define 'N/A' (not applicable) labels.

## DATA ENTRY

Data entry can occur live while video is being captured onto the computer disk. The different software platforms operate in distinct data capture modes as well as analysis modes. For example, the same Category Set in Focus X2 is used in both logging mode and review mode. Similarly, the Code Window of sportscode can be used to enter labels when in coding mode or labelling mode. Irrespective of the package being used there are common principles of live data entry systems that need to be implemented. The first of these is that the system is usable in real-time typically requiring well trained users and the live part of the system is restricted to the most critical events. The use of hot-keys is also recommended for live systems. These are keys of the keyboard that are assigned to on-screen buttons representing events and labels. The user can press a key of the keyboard quicker than using the mouse to click on an on-screen button. The pre-roll and post-roll (or lead and lag times) that are used with many event types need to consider that the users will not have been able to pause the video at the exact point of the event before entering data for the event. The match video is being captured live and cannot be paused. Therefore, events may be entered slightly after the point in time at which they actually occur. It is also useful to have an 'error' event! Where the user is aware they have keyed in something wrong, they may not be able to correct the event while further events are occurring in the match that need to be recorded. The sportscode package does allow events in the timeline to have incorrect labels removed and correct labels added while the video is still capturing. However, this would typically require some interruption to the match for the operator to do this. Therefore, a simple error button can be pressed (the author uses the space bar of the keyboard for this) which marks the position of any errors made allowing them to be identified and corrected shortly after the match has finished.

Focus Voice (within the Focus package) is an example of data entry using voice recognition software. Cort (2006) found a high level of reliability of word recognition by Voice Focus. However, Cort's (2006) study only looked at errors between the words spoken by the human coder and the words recorded by Focus Voice. There, may be additional errors in the verbal coding of behaviour that result from voice strain or motor delays when verbally coding. There may also be perceptual errors made by observers that are not accounted for by Cort's (2006) method. The data for some live systems can be captured separately to the video with these two types of data being integrated and synchronised later. Pocket Focus allows users to enter data using the Category Set on a handheld computer. The data can then be linked to the match video later.

Some systems involve a combination of live and post-match data entry. This is certainly the case where all of the data required cannot be entered live during the match. The key events that are needed to produce information shortly after the match would be entered live with other data being entered post match. One strategy is to ensure all events are tagged live and then any additional labels (in sportscode) or values of categories not entered live (in Focus X2) are entered afterwards. This can be very efficient because the user does not need to watch the whole match again because the areas where further data entry are needed are already identified by coded events.

Post-match labelling of events can be done very efficiently using the graphical user interface. sportscode, for example, provides a labelling mode that allows users to repeatedly review event clips entering any label buttons using the Code Windows that apply. In Focus X2, users can change values from defaults to the correct values within the Event List using drop-down menus.

## ANALYSIS FACILITIES

In sportscode, there is a clear distinction between events and data labels. In Focus X2, on the other hand, an event record contains a value for each

computerised performance analysis systems

of the categories in the Category Set. While events in Focus X2 are timed on one category and logged on another (these two categories could be the same), there is no distinction made between different types of event beyond the values used. The main quantitative analysis feature of commercial video analysis packages is the cross-tabulation of values. In Focus X2, for example, one category is selected as the rows of the cross-tabulation and another category is selected as columns. The cross-tabulated frequencies for these two categories can be derived from all logged events or from events satisfying criteria that are specified in the Category Set during review mode. Consider Figure 7.3 where the greyed values of categories have been selected. Here we are only interested in the passes made by members of our own team (Us). So all players, pitch areas and outcomes are included, but there is only one event type (pass) and one team (Us) selected. Having selected these criteria, only the events satisfying the criteria appear in the Event List. If we cross-tabulate player with outcome, when these criteria are specified, we will see the number of successful and unsuccessful passes made by each player on our team. This can be done for other event types or combinations of event types.

The Matrix facility of sportscode cross-tabulates events with value labels to show the frequency distribution of labels for each event type. The rows of the Matrix are events and the columns of the Matrix are value labels. The timeline contains a row for each event type that shows the instances of the event type that have been recorded. After data entry, further rows can be created in the timeline by AND-ing or OR-ing existing rows together. When two rows are AND-ed together, a new row is created containing an instance for each period of time where instances are recorded in both rows. Where the durations of the two existing instances

| Category | Values | | | | | |
|---|---|---|---|---|---|---|
| Event type | Pass | Shot | Tackle | Keeping | Restart | Interception |
| Team | Us | | | Opposition | | |
| Player | 1 | 2 | 3 | 4 | 5 | 6 | 7 | 8 | 9 | 10 | 11 |
| Pitch area | DL | DC | DR | ML | MC | MR | AL | AC | AR |
| Outcome | Successful | | | | Unsuccessful | | |

Figure 7.3 Selecting event criteria in a Focus X2 category set

overlap, the instance created in the new row has a duration that is common to the two existing instances. This starts at the latest start point of the two existing instances and finishes at the earliest end point of the two existing instances. When two rows are OR-ed together, a new row is created containing instances at the times where there are instances in one or other of the existing rows. Where instances overlap in the two existing rows, the new row combines them within an instance that uses the earliest start point of the two original instances and the latest end point of the two existing instances. For example, we might not just want to know the number of passes made in a given area and the number of passes that are successful; we might also want to know the number of successful passes made in the given area of the field.

The Matrices and full Event Lists recorded for matches can be exported for further analysis in spreadsheet packages such as Microsoft Excel. These spreadsheets can be pre-programmed to calculate summary percentages and ratios of interest and can be used for successive matches by simply pasting in the exported data for newly coded matches.

**Interactive video feedback**

The main purpose of general purpose video analysis packages is to allow flexible interactive video feedback. The storage of video on random access devices, such as computer disks, allows the packages to efficiently access the required video frames given the video times of these frames. The Matrices of sportscode show the frequencies of events where different labels have been included. Directly clicking on these frequencies within Matrices displays the video sequences in question. The process in Focus X2 is that criteria of interest can be selected reducing the number of events shown in the Event List. Video sequences for events in the Event List satisfying the specified criteria can then be displayed. The packages simply look up the events of interest, determining their start and end times, any pre- and post-roll times to be used and play the appropriate video frames.

**Creating highlight movies**

The advantages of interactive video feedback are that the analyst does not need to spend additional time producing movie files for debriefings

computerised performance analysis systems

and the video sequences can be displayed by the package as soon as the match has finished. Indeed, in some packages, video sequences of recorded events can be displayed while the match video is still being captured. The disadvantage of using interactive video feedback is that coaches and analysts may not have selected the best events to show and the process of selecting and replaying video clips can interrupt briefings. A further disadvantage is that coaches may not have the video analysis packages installed on their computers and rely on analysts and the analysts' computers to display video clips. Therefore, highlights movies may need to be produced for briefings or debriefings. These movies can be played using standard media playing packages available on most computers. Producing a highlights movie involves selecting events of interest, previewing the related video sequences, selecting the best clips to display and then saving these in a standalone movie file. Some packages allow titles, annotations and notes to be added to such movies, for example the Movie Organiser facility in sportscode permits such editing. Other packages require movies to be saved as standalone movie files and then further edited using general purpose video editing software such as iMovie (Apple Inc., Cupertino, CA). Once the highlights video has been created, it can be used efficiently within briefing/debriefing meetings to provide feedback to players. The disadvantage of producing standalone highlights movies is that it takes time and can tie up the analyst's machine while video files are being saved.

## GENERAL PURPOSE ANALYSIS WITHOUT VIDEO

Visual BASIC data entry interfaces can be developed to populate Microsoft Excel spreadsheets or Microsoft Access databases. The data entry interfaces can set up groups of buttons that can be used in a similar way to the Category Sets of Focus X2. Once the match event data have been recorded, they can be analysed in an efficient manner permitting the benefits of both sequential data and frequency data. This is an advantage over manual systems where the analyst often has to make a choice between using a sequential system or a frequency table. If an Event List is stored in a relational database, standard database querying can be used to filter events providing frequencies of interest. If the data are stored in an Excel spreadsheet then pivot tables can be used to cross-tabulate sets of variables showing frequencies of different combinations of values. The main disadvantage of such systems is that there is no video component and, therefore, such systems are typically used in academic research rather than within coaching.

## SPECIAL PURPOSE MATCH ANALYSIS SYSTEMS

### Rationale for special purpose systems

The difference between a general purpose match analysis package and a special purpose match analysis system is that the general purpose package can be tailored for use with any sport while the special purpose package is used with a specific sport. The general purpose match analysis packages provide video tagging, statistical feedback and flexible interactive review of video sequences. This leads to the question as to why special purpose systems are needed. The rationale for special purpose systems has been made by considering their relative advantages and disadvantages over general purpose systems (Williams, 2004). A general purpose system provides a standard interface and set of processes for capture, analysis and presentation of data. The functions can be too restricted for the analyses required in some sports. There may also be features of general purpose systems that are not used by some users who work with a single sport. While the general purpose package may provide everything that is required for analysis of the given sport, the additional unused facilities of the package still contribute to its cost. The costs not only relate to the general purpose packages themselves but also to the computer hardware that is required to use the packages. Williams (2004) also discussed the limitations of standardised interfaces and limited capture options of general purpose packages.

Williams (2004) listed several additional advantages of special purpose systems besides overcoming the limitations of using general purpose packages. Sports specific data structures can be used within special purpose systems to promote efficient data storage and retrieval for the specific analysis functions required. Special purpose packages can be developed to use sports specific output formats, such as wagon wheel charts in cricket. Such formats are commonly used and well understood by coaches and journalists covering the specific sport. Behaviour in some sports follows 'match syntax'. Syntax in linguistics is the set of rules and principles governing the structure of sentences. In computer programming languages and spreadsheet programming, such rules are also used to help the computer understand the program instruction code allowing it to be executed. In sports performance, there are behaviours where event sequences or data entered about events have to fit within allowable patterns for the sport. For example, in tennis, a point is made up of the serve, possible additional shots and ends on a winner or error. A tennis analysis system could be developed to enforce allowable ordering of events and event data during data entry. There may be some events that occur that require specific additional data not required by other event types. The event performed may restrict the set of event types that can happen next. Special purpose systems can be developed in a way that interfaces restrict data entry options to only those that are valid in given match states. There are specific aspects of sports that are so unique to those sports that general purpose packages cannot be expected to provide all of these. For example, the challenge system in tennis requires analysis systems to be able to change the outcome of a point due to the challenge or ensure the point does not contribute to the score. Functions to process data in specific ways required by the sport can also be included in special purpose systems. When using general purpose packages, such processing often requires data to be exported into spreadsheet packages for additional processing. Data consistency checks are also possible within special purpose systems. These are more to do with semantics than syntax. In linguistics, semantics is concerned with the meaning of sentences. A sentence could be syntactically correct but with semantic errors. In sports performance analysis, an example of a semantic error would be where we have entered that a tennis point has been won by the serving player with a winner and that there was an even number of shots including the serve. This is not possible, because shots alternate between the two players and so for the server to win the point with a winner there would need to have been an odd number of shots. Special purpose systems can be programmed to spot such errors and prompt users to provide correct information. In this tennis example, the correct data could be that the receiver won the point with a winner, that the server won the point with an opponent error or that there were an odd number of shots rather than an even number of shots.

There are also disadvantages of using special purpose systems. They need to be developed and this can require time and be costly. Special purpose systems may not have as professionally produced help files and user manuals as general purpose packages. This is often the case where a special purpose system is developed by an analyst solely for their own personal use. Maintenance of special purpose systems is also an issue as users may prefer to continue using existing versions of systems rather than upgrading them to take advantage of hardware improvements.

## Single user systems

This chapter distinguishes between two broad types of special purpose system: systems that are developed for particular users and commercial special purpose match analysis packages that are available for purchase and use by users in given sports and the media. An example of a system developed for particular users is the system developed by Williams (2004) for use in his own PhD study. Williams (2004) was undertaking a scientific research project into the effect of rule changes on rugby union performance. There was no need for interactive video feedback as the system was not intended for use in coaching environments. The areas of the sport that were of interest to the study were represented in an entity relationship model that defined the database component of the system. The system allowed game events to be entered into the database and individual game reports to be produced. The outputs included timings for ball in play, possession and territory. The study required Williams to apply his abilities in system development using Visual BASIC and empirical research in sports science.

## Prozone MatchViewer

Special purpose systems have been developed commercially for use in coaching. The Prozone company is best known for its player tracking system, Prozone3, that has been used in soccer. Prozone also provides a soccer specific match analysis system that is used to analyse on-the-ball action. The system is called Prozone MatchViewer and is affordable to amateur teams while also being relevant to the requirements of expert coaches at elite levels of soccer. Unlike Prozone3, MatchViewer does not need to be installed permanently at a single stadium. There are five main variables recorded for each event; event type, time of the event, player 1 involved, player 2 involved (if applicable) and pitch location (recorded on a bird's eye image of the pitch). Frequencies of on-the-ball events are provided as general match statistics. Player specific match statistics include passing, shooting, goalkeeping and crossing statistics. Event Lists

158

can be produced for individual player contributions or for a team as a whole. The pitch diagram is a type of scatter plot but is interactive allowing direct selection of events with the mouse to activate video replay of those events. The system is flexible allowing time periods for events of interest and other criteria to be specified.

## Special purpose cricket systems

Petersen and Dawson (2013) listed the special purpose packages used in cricket; these are Feedback Cricket (Feedback Sport, Christchurch, New Zealand), Crickstat (CSIR, Pretoria, South Africa), The Cricket Analyst program (Fairplay Sports, Jindalee, Queensland, Australia) and Optiplay Cricket (CSIR, Pretoria, South Africa).

Crickstat DV (CSIR, Pretoria, South Africa) integrates match video, objective data and data imported from other systems such as Hawkeye (Hawkeye Innovations, Basingstoke, UK). Information about match and venue settings can be entered at the beginning of match analysis together with details of the teams competing. The visual outputs of the system include wagon wheel diagrams which can be viewed from multiple perspectives, three dimensional views of wickets displaying information about deliveries, 'worm charts' showing cumulative runs made and 'Manhattan charts' displaying run frequencies for the overs played. Information relating to batting partnerships is available together with video sequence output.

CSIR has developed Optiplay Cricket to replace Crickstat. Like many commercial products, there are different versions incorporating different features aimed at different market sectors including academic and team use. The 'Scorer' version of the system provides basic analysis of batting and bowling including worm charts and Manhattans charts, which are histograms of runs accumulated in an over. The version of the system with the greatest functionality is Optiplay Elite which includes capture and tagging of video footage as well as flexible review of video sequences by specifying criteria of interest.

## IBM's analysis of Grand Slam tennis

There are special purpose systems for various sports used to provide summary statistics on media channels (Kirkbride, 2013b). These include statistics for international soccer matches that are provided by FIFA's (Fédération Internationale de Football Association) website (www.fifa.com) and the IRB's (International Rugby Board) website (www.irb.com). Other organisations analyse soccer matches providing data on a commercial basis, for example Optasports (www.optasports.com). This section of the chapter discusses the statistics provided on the official websites of the four Grand Slam tennis tournaments. The statistics are 'presented' by IBM and have been used in television coverage of matches as well as academic research (O'Donoghue, 2002). The following statistics are provided for each player's performance in each set as well as for the match as a whole:

- The number of first serve and second serve points played and won and the percentage of points won on each serve.
- The number of receiving points played and won and the percentage of points won when receiving.
- The number of aces and double faults that are played.
- The number of net points played and won and the percentage of net points that are won.
- The number of break points played and won and the percentage of break points that are won.
- The number of winners and unforced errors played.
- The speed of the fastest serve, the mean speed of first serves and the mean speed of second serves.
- Serve direction statistics: the number of points played and won when serving to the left, middle and right of the deuce and advantage courts on first and second serves. The serve direction statistics also include the number of aces and speed statistics for serves played in each direction to each service court on first and second serve.
- Rally statistics: frequencies of approach shots, drop shots, ground strokes, lobs, overhead shots, passing shots and volleys.

The serve speed statistics are only provided for matches played on courts where a radar gun is installed. Some of the raw data required for the other statistics are gathered by trained observers using palm top computers. There are other matches where the statistics only cover points played and won without any details about net points.

The Slam Tracker facility provided on the tournament websites provides temporal information by showing sequences of points in various forms.

computerised performance analysis systems

A 'Momentum graph' shows where each player is winning points. Points on the momentum chart can be clicked with the mouse to obtain further information about them. Particular events such as aces or double faults can be superimposed on this chart. The Slam Tracker facility also provides a list of text details about the points in the match. For, example these are the details recorded for 2013 US Open final between Novak Djokovic and Rafael Nadal:

R. Nadal loses the point with a forehand forced error: 15–0
N. Djokovic loses the point with a backhand volley forced error: 15–15
R. Nadal loses the point with a backhand unforced error: 30–15
N. Djokovic loses the point with a backhand unforced error: 30–30
R. Nadal loses the point with a forehand forced error: 40–30
N. Djokovic wins the point with an ace: 0–0
N. Djokovic loses the point with a backhand unforced error: 0–15
N. Djokovic loses the point with a backhand unforced error: 0–30

.
.
.
.
.

This type of information can be analysed using the text processing functions of Microsoft Excel as described by O'Donoghue and Holmes (2015: Chapter 3). The validity of the information provided on the Grand Slam tournament websites is evidenced from its sustained use in broadcast coverage and coaching. Commentators understand the statistics well enough to make meaningful assessments about the states of matches. Indeed players and coaches also understand the statistics. When Laura Robson was interviewed after her third-round defeat by Li Na in the 2013 US Open, she was asked what three things she would like to improve over the 12 months to the 2014 US Open (Sky, 2013). She responded with two areas; a better first serve percentage and fewer unforced errors. Irrespective the validity of the data or the purpose of their use, whether for coaching, media or scientific research purposes, the data have to be reliable. This applies to any data that are being used from secondary sources such as official tournament internet sites. There is evidence that the first and second serve statistics (Knight and O'Donoghue, 2012), serve direction statistics (O'Donoghue, 2009) and net points (O'Donoghue and Holmes, 2015: Chapter 9) are sufficiently reliable.

## SUMMARY

Computerised systems are now commonplace in sports performance analysis and range from the use of general purpose data analysis packages such as Excel and Access with Visual BASIC interfaces to sophisticated video analysis packages that can be tailored for use with multiple sports. The commercially available general purpose video analysis packages typically come in versions suitable for different market sectors ranging from entry level analysis to elite level systems. This has made feedback technology available to coaches and athletes at club level as well as to international squads with support teams. Despite the cost effectiveness and flexibility of these packages, there are still niche areas of the sports performance analysis market where special purpose systems are used providing sport specific data representation and processing capability. These systems include sports specific functions that could not be expected within a general purpose package that needs to provide common core functionality to suit a large number of sport types.

# CHAPTER 8

## WORKED EXAMPLES OF COMPUTERISED PERFORMANCE ANALYSIS SYSTEMS

### INTRODUCTION

This chapter will take the two examples used in Chapter 6 and show how they can be implemented in commercial match analysis packages. The tennis example illustrates the use of the Matrix facility to produce frequencies of different combinations of serves and outcomes. The soccer possession analysis example illustrates how the three types of system described in Chapter 5 (scatter plot, frequency table and sequential system) can be combined when using a commercial match analysis package. The chapter uses a third example of a computerised system which is for time-motion analysis. This system is used in Chapter 9 to discuss reliability assessment and in Chapter 10 to discuss report writing.

The tennis and soccer possession examples are not covered in as much depth as they were in Chapter 6. This is because a lot of the decisions about what events and modifying information to use were discussed in Chapter 6 meaning that the current chapter can concentrate on the process of implementing such systems using commercial match analysis packages. This raises a more fundamental point which is that analysts developing systems using commercial packages should consider system requirements, outputs, inputs, data stores and functions before entering a commercial match analysis package. This is also a reason why computerised match analysis is typically covered in sports performance analysis degree programmes after students have mastered some basic system design skills during the development of manual systems.

## TENNIS EXAMPLE

### The problem

We wish to develop and use a computerised version of the tennis system described in Chapter 6 so that we can have a chronological list of point records and the ability to determine frequencies for different variables and combinations of variables. Recall that we had six variables in the manual version of the system:

- Set (1st, 2nd, 3rd, 4th or 5th).
- Service (1st or 2nd serve).
- Service court (deuce or advantage).
- Area of the service court served to (left, middle or right third).
- Type of serve (flat, slice or kick).
- Outcome of point (Won or Lost).

The manual system addressed set by using a different form for each set. We will add an additional variable to the computerised system which is player. Player was a variable in the manual version of the system but, like set, required a separate copy of the data collection form to be used for each player.

### An initial solution

This chapter will describe two computerised versions of the system, both of which are implemented in sportscode. These are possible solutions and there are others that readers may feel are better. The purpose of the first solution is to highlight usability problems in computerised systems that can be overcome through improved design. Computerised packages allow systems to be created, checked and revised within a rapid proto-typing approach where difficulties experienced using early versions can be overcome when amending the system.

Figure 8.1 shows the first attempt for the system; this is the Code Window. The grey buttons are simply titles for other button clusters. The buttons with a diamond in the top right-hand corner are event buttons that are used to record events occurring within the timeline. Recall from Chapter 7 that a timeline in sportscode is associated with the match video

# 164

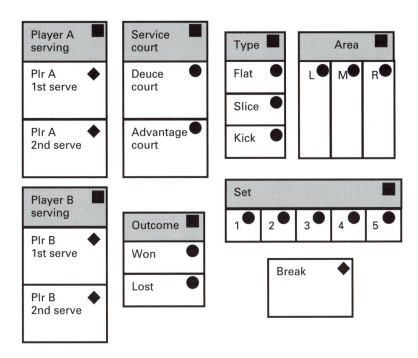

**Figure 8.1** An initial computerised version of the tennis serve system

allowing the video to be indexed or tagged with timed events. There are events representing points where Player A and Player B take first serves and second serves as well as an event type representing inter-point breaks. These event buttons are exclusively linked meaning that when a new event, such as an inter-point break commences, any other event that is currently active is deactivated. Therefore, we will only see one event having been recorded at any time in the timeline. Where a player takes a first serve and a second serve within the same point, both events remain in the timeline. However, it is only the second serve where event labels will be entered if the serve is in. Where a 'let' occurs on either first or second serve, the user can choose whether or not to hit the Tab key to end the event for the let serve and then enter a new event for the serve that is going to count. Doing the latter means that the video clip for the serve will not include the let serve. Some users may prefer that the let serve is included as well as the serve that counts. If this is the case, they simply should not press the Tab key when the let occurs. There is a lead time of 3 seconds for the four different service events which allows the service motion to be shown fully on the video clips of points. This is preferable to video sequences commencing at the point the server strikes the ball. At the end of the point, there will be a short period where label buttons are entered before the user activates the 'Break' event for inter-point breaks. When the user presses this button depends on how much they wish to include on the video clip for the point after it has ended.

The buttons with circles in the top right-hand corner are data labels. These allow modifier information to be included within event instances in the timeline. The data labels include service court served to, area of the service court that is served to, type of serve and outcome of the point. The set label buttons are entered at the end of the match. The user simply puts sportscode into label mode, selects the series of events that occur in the first set and then press the button '1' to include this label in the events. The same is done for the remaining sets in the match. Some users trying this system will find it annoying that they enter 'Won' or 'Lost' at the end of the point and yet still have to enter 'Break'. This is a fair point! An alternative might be to activate the 'Break' button when either 'Won' or 'Lost' is entered. Users are welcome to try such a solution as an exercise.

Once a match has been tagged using this system, it can be analysed. The default Matrix will not provide information on the different combinations of services, service courts, serve types, areas of service courts and point outcomes that the manual version of the system provided. To produce this type of information we need to create additional rows in the time-line and the Matrix needs to be extended with columns for combinations of label values. We will already have four rows in the timeline:

- Player A 1st Serve
- Player A 2nd Serve
- Player B 1st Serve
- Player B 2nd Serve

A new row is created in the timeline using **Row → Create New Row**. A popup window appears where we enter the name of the new row (for example Player A Serve), the two rows to be combined (for example Player A 1st Serve and Player A 2nd Serve) and the type of operator used to combine them (for example OR). When events are OR-ed together in the time line, there is an instance in the new row at any point in time when there is an instance in either or both of the two original rows being combined. One thing to take note of is that if lead times are too long, then there may be occasions where two different events are combined into a single event in the new row where they overlap. This is not likely to happen in this tennis system because points alternate with inter-point breaks. Where instances of first and second serves to a given service court are merged, there will be overlap but this does not matter so much because there will only be one set of labels for the second serve in such cases. In systems that students are developing for other sports, they should consider events that may be merged, the lead times and lag times involved as well as events that are mutually exclusively. The newly created rows within the timeline are:

■ Player A Serve (which combines the player's first and second serve points).
■ Player B Serve (which combines the player's first and second serve points).

The Matrix is extended to include columns combining labels. Initially, the Matrix will contain single labels:

■ Deuce court
■ Advantage court
■ Flat
■ Slice
■ Kick
■ L
■ M
■ R
■ Won
■ Lost
■ 1
■ 2
■ 3
■ 4
■ 5

We can now extend the Matrix to include combinations of labels, for example we might want to know about points won when serving to the deuce court. This is done by clicking the 'Deuce court' button with the

CTRL key held down. A menu appears and we choose to duplicate the 'Deuce court' column. The duplicate column of the Matrix is dragged to the location where we require it. We can now add 'Won' to the column and choose a combination operator such as AND operator; thus the column becomes 'Deuce court AND Won'. If we are just interested in statistics, we do not need 'Deuce court AND Lost' because the frequency of 'Deuce court AND Won' labels can be expressed as a percentage of all 'Deuce' points. However, if we might be interested in seeing video clips of points lost when serving to the deuce court then we should include 'Deuce court AND Lost'. The combined labels include:

- Deuce court AND Won
- Deuce court AND Lost
- Advantage court AND Won
- Advantage court AND Lost
- Flat AND Won
- Flat AND Lost
- Slice AND Won
- Slice AND Lost
- Kick AND Won
- Kick AND Lost
- L AND Won
- L AND Lost
- M AND Won
- M AND Lost
- R AND Won
- R AND Lost
- Deuce court AND Flat AND Won
- Deuce court AND Flat AND Lost
- Deuce court AND Slice AND Won
- Deuce court AND Slice AND Lost
- Deuce court AND Kick AND Won
- Deuce court AND Kick AND Lost
- Advantage court AND Flat AND Won
- Advantage court AND Flat AND Lost
- Advantage court AND Slice AND Won
- Advantage court AND Slice AND Lost
- Advantage court AND Kick AND Won.
- Advantage court AND Kick AND Lost
- . . . and many more

168

There are a great deal of combinations of two, three, four or all five of the two service courts, three serve types, three areas of the service court, two point outcomes and five sets. Therefore, we may wish to limit the number of combinations to those of most relevance to the coach. The extended Matrix will have many columns. Therefore, an alternative is to have more events and fewer labels to make the resulting Matrix squarer. An example of such a Code Window is shown in Figure 8.2. This will have eight rows for the eight different conditions of player, service court, and whether the serve is a first or second serve:

- Plr A 1st Serve Deuce Court
- Plr A 2nd Serve Deuce Court
- Plr A 1st Serve Adv Court
- Plr A 2nd Serve Adv Court
- Plr B 1st Serve Deuce Court
- Plr B 2nd Serve Deuce Court
- Plr B 1st Serve Adv Court
- Plr B 2nd Serve Adv Court

The additional rows to be created are:

- Plr A Deuce Court
- Plr A Adv Court
- Plr A 1st Serve
- Plr A 2nd Serve
- Plr A All Serves
- Plr B Deuce Court
- Plr B Adv Court
- Plr B 1st Serve
- Plr B 2nd Serve
- Plr B All Serves

There is a third way of producing these additional rows while the events are being entered. This is to have these higher order serve events within the Code Window and automatically activated by the event buttons shown in Figure 8.3. Thus when 'Plr A 1st Serve Deuce Court' is entered, it automatically activates 'Plr A Deuce Court' and 'Plr A 1st Serve'. Either one of these events can then automatically activate 'Plr A All Serves'.

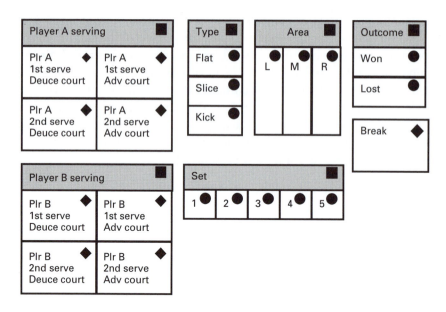

**Figure 8.2** A second solution to the tennis serve example

We could have done something similar with labels having nine label buttons 'L Flat', 'L Slice', 'L Kick', 'M Flat', 'M Slice', 'M Kick', 'R Flat', 'R Slice' and 'R Kick' which could then activate higher order labels for the three serve types and the three areas of the service court. An added advantage of such an approach is that it means we only have to click on one label button rather than two buttons to enter type of serve and area of court. If students are using versions of sportscode that do not permit the Matrix to be extended then this might be the better solution. This third solution produces higher order events using activation links as shown in Figure 8.3. For example, where the user clicks on the event 'Plr A 1st Serve Deuce Court', activation links can automatically start higher order events such as 'Plr A 1st Serve' and 'Plr A Deuce Court'. One of these could then activate an even higher order event 'Plr A Serve'. The advantage of doing this is that the timeline and Matrix will already have rows for combined factor events such as 'Plr A 1st Serve Deuce Court' as well as the higher order events. The disadvantages are that the time-line contains many more rows and if a mistake is made entering a value label, then this will have to be corrected in the combined factor event

170

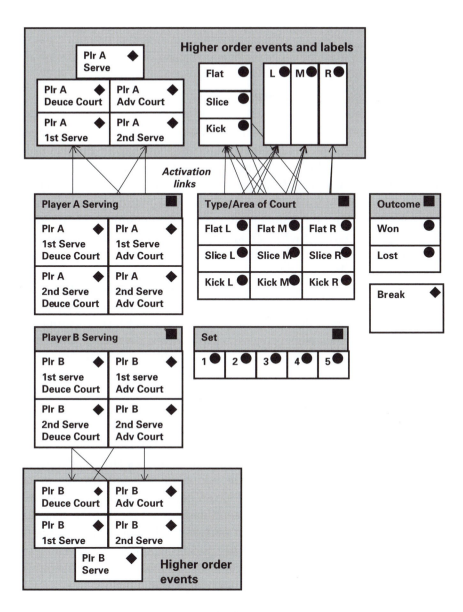

**Figure 8.3** Using activation links to higher order events

instances concerned and any higher order event instances that were activated. For example, if we entered the label 'Flat L' mistakenly rather than 'Flat M' during a 'Plr A 1st Serve Deuce Court' then the label would need to be corrected in the higher order 'Plr A 1st Serve', 'Plr A Deuce Court' and 'Plr A Serve' events as well.

## SOCCER POSSESSION EXAMPLE

Consider the soccer possession analysis system that was used as an example of manual notation in Chapter 6. In the current chapter, this example is used to illustrate the development of a computerised match analysis system using packages such as sportscode and Nacsport. The particular version of the system illustrated here does not require possessions to alternate. Therefore, the outcome of a possession could be 'Retained' if the next possession was a free kick, corner or throw in, for example, for the team in possession of the ball. The possession events are exclusively linked so that when a new possession starts, any currently recording possession is terminated. Figure 8.4 shows that the sportscode implementation uses a code button for each of the possession types when performed by each of the two teams ('Us' and 'Them'). Duplicating the event buttons for each team is necessary to ensure a new possession event starts if one team had a possession starting with a tackle and then the other team takes possession with a tackle. If we simply had a tackle code button and used value labels for the two teams we would need to use the Tab key to end one tackle event and then use the tackle code button to start the next possession. If we simply press that tackle code button applying the label for one team and then press the tackle button again applying the label for the other team, there will be a single possession event having started with a tackle which both teams appear to be performing. Using separate sets of seven code buttons for possessions performed by 'Us' and 'Them' has an added advantage that the user can enter possession type and the team performing it with a single click of the mouse. There are activation links to higher order possession type events as well as possessions performed by 'Us' and 'Them'. Value labels are used to record pitch areas and possession outcomes.

The computerised implementation allows more flexibility and efficient analysis than the manual version covered in Chapter 6. A full Event List can be exported and matrices of events and data label combinations can be displayed and exported. A similar implementation of the system in the Nacsport package allows a combination of scatterplots, a sequential system and frequency tables to be used. These were the three different

worked examples of computerised systems

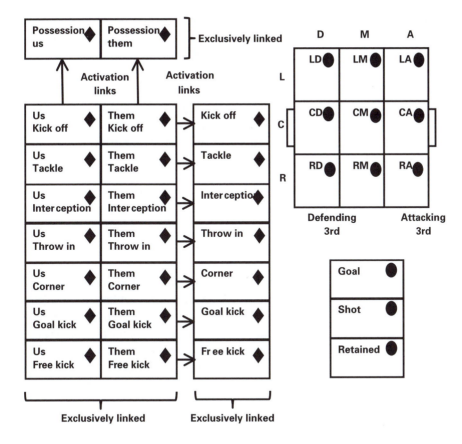

Figure 8.4 sportscode version of the soccer possession example

types of manual notation system covered in Chapter 5 where analysts often had to make choices between them due to their relative advantages and disadvantages. When using a commercial match analysis package to implement a system, we do not suffer the disadvantages that exist in manual systems. We can use an Event List (sequential system) and very efficiently produce a Matrix (this is essentially a frequency table). This is because the chronological Event List is stored and can be exported, data matrices and sub-matrices can be produced immediately by the computer and event locations can be entered on an image of the playing surface. A JPEG image can be used to represent the playing surface with event locations recorded using the image. This allows the locations of different types of event to be shown, with the option to use lines to link sequences of events in chronological order on the playing surface image. In the soccer possession analysis example, the locations of the events that started the possessions could be entered, for example tackles, interceptions, free kicks, etc. This does not show the full path of the ball during the possession but a finer grain system could record individual passes. A major benefit of the computerised systems is that they permit video sequences of events satisfying criteria of interest to be replayed very efficiently or included in highlights movies.

## WORK-RATE ANALYSIS EXAMPLE

### Two-movement system

Work-rate analysis, or time-motion analysis, is used as an example in Chapter 9 for reliability evaluation. Work-rate analysis is a good example to use in coursework exercises because locomotive movement is a general concept in sport and does not require students to understand details of rules, tactics and techniques in specific sports. Therefore, work-rate analysis is used as an example of reliability evaluation in the second coursework done in the Level 5 Sports Performance Analysis module at the author's university. The write up of the work-rate analysis exercise is covered in Chapter 10. Unlike the first coursework, where the students develop a system for a sport of their choice, the second coursework requires the students to evaluate the reliability of already developed systems. One example of such a system is the two-movement work-rate analysis system where the activity of a player under observation is classified as 'work' or 'rest'. This is done subjectively with operators classifying any movement that they perceive to require high intensity effort as 'work'. All remaining low or moderate intensity activity is classified as 'rest'. Figure 8.5 shows that the system can be implemented in sportscode using two exclusively linked events; 'Work' and 'Rest'. Analysis of data entered using this system determines the number of work and rest periods, the mean duration of work and rest periods as well as the percentage of observation time that the player spent performing work. The number of work and rest periods should differ by no more than one because these activities alternate. The percentage of time spent performing rest activities is not required because this will be 100 minus the percentage of time spent performing work. This information can be

worked examples of computerised systems

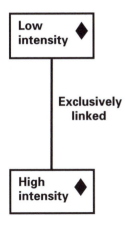

**Figure 8.5** Two-movement work-rate analysis system

obtained by simply exporting an instance frequency report. This can be exported as an Excel spreadsheet which will contain the frequency, total time, percentage time and mean duration of each event type (work and rest). If more detailed information is needed about the number of work (or rest) periods of different duration sub-ranges then users may need to examine an exported Event List or use a Statistical Window.

The kappa value used to evaluate reliability of time-motion analysis systems is covered in Chapter 9. In order to produce kappa, we need to determine the amount of time where two independent observations agreed on the activity being performed by the player. We will have two timeline files to compare (say t1 and t2). Both of the timelines will have used the same Code Window and thus have the same row names ('Work' and 'Rest'). It is necessary to distinguish between the instances recorded in two observations when the timelines are merged for the purpose of reliability assessment. This is done by making a copy of one of the time-lines where we can use different row names. For example we could make a copy of the file t2 and call it t2copy. We select both rows in the file t2copy ('Work' and 'Rest') and duplicate them using **Rows → Duplicate selected rows**. This creates two new rows ('Work[1]' and 'Rest[1]') containing the same instances as the original rows. We can now delete the original two rows from t2copy. We now merge the rows within t1 and t2copy into a merged timeline which we call tmerged. This is done by opening the timeline files t1 and t2copy and selecting both rows in each file. We then use **File → Merge timeline windows** which creates a new timeline with all four rows copied into it which we save as merged. This is used to determine the amount of observation time where the observers agreed that work was being performed and the amount of observation time where the observers agreed that rest was being performed. Consider the rows representing where the two observers have recorded work ('Work' and 'Work[1]'). We create a new row containing instances where the two observers agree that the player was performing Work using **Row → Create new row** which causes a popup window to appear. In this popup window, we advise that the new row will be called 'Work_agreed', selecting the rows 'Work' and 'Work[1]' and applying the AND operator. This new row ('Work_agreed') only contains instances of work where there is some overlap between the instances recorded by the two observers.

**Seven-movement system**

Figure 8.6 shows an alternative work-rate analysis system where movement is classified into seven movements. Four of these are low intensity activities; stationary, walking, backing and jogging. The remaining three activities are counted as high intensity activity; running (which includes sprinting), shuffling and game related activity. The individual movement classes are exclusively linked so that when a new movement instance commences, any current movement instance is terminated. The seven-movement types also activate higher order 'work' and 'rest' behaviours. The frequency, mean duration and percentage time spent performing each movement type can be obtained by exporting an instance frequency report. The proportion of observation time where two observations agree on the activity being performed is done in a similar way to that described for the two-movement system. The difference here is that there are two sets of seven movement types and hence a set of seven merged rows; one for each movement activity.

**SUMMARY**

This chapter has shown how the tennis and soccer possession analysis systems covered in Chapter 6 can be implemented using commercial

worked examples of computerised systems

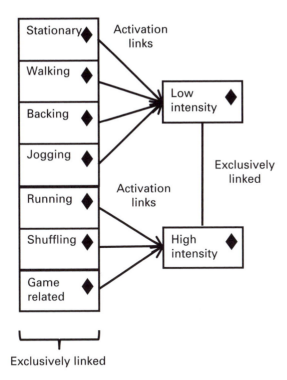

**Figure 8.6** Seven movement work-rate analysis system

generic performance analysis systems. While using manual notation often forces us to choose between using a sequential system and a frequency table, computerised systems give us the best of all words with the chronologically ordered list of events being preserved and a much more efficient way of producing event frequency summaries as data matrices. Where systems, such as Nacsport, allow event locations to be entered onto pitch diagrams, we can also combine the benefits of scatter plots with those of sequential systems and frequency tables. The computerised systems also have the ability to automatically produce higher order event information through the use of activation links. The chapter also covers two versions of a work-rate analysis system that are used to discuss reliability in Chapter 9.

# CHAPTER 9

## RELIABILITY TESTING

### INTRODUCTION

This chapter initially discusses what reliability is and its relation to objectivity and validity before covering reliability statistics used in sports performance analysis. The chapter uses the tennis serving and soccer possession systems described in Chapters 6 and 8 to illustrate how percentage error and kappa can be calculated. Kappa can be used where we have a sequential system with a chronological list of event records. Kappa cannot be used where we only have tallies recorded in a frequency table. However, percentage error can be used in such situations. The chapter uses time-motion analysis to illustrate how kappa can also be used to assess the reliability of continuous time data. The time-motion analysis system is used to consider reliability levels in relation to the goals of performance analysis tasks. A final example of 800m running is used to illustrate how to determine the reliability of ratio scale numeric variables such as split times. This example illustrates the use of mean absolute error and correlation coefficients.

### VALIDITY, OBJECTIVITY AND RELIABILITY

#### Validity

This section of the chapter distinguishes the measurement issues of validity, objectivity and reliability with respect to sports performance analysis. The relationships between these measurement concepts are covered using the example of the computerised scoring system in amateur boxing. Validity was discussed during Chapter 3 when performance indicators were introduced. Performance indicators must be valid and represent some relevant and important aspect of sports performance. If a variable is a meaningless statistic that nobody understands and nobody cares about, it cannot be valid. The value of a performance indicator needs to be understandable so that coaches and players can make decisions using its value. Therefore, analysts and coaches must understand the meaning of performance indicators, their definitions and the ranges of values that are considered to be high, low and average. All performance indicators need to be valid, but there may be other valid variables that do not have all of the qualities of performance indicators. Therefore, valid variables that are relevant and important should not automatically be termed performance indicators.

Validity can also apply to entire systems and the sets of information they produce. Content validity is the extent to which a set of variables covers the relevant and important aspects of performance in a given sport. Content validity can also apply to sports performance profiles which are collections of variables representing different aspects of performance.

**Objectivity**

Objectivity was covered in Chapter 2 when qualitative and quantitative data were being compared. Objectivity means that there is some definition or guidance for measuring a sports performance variable so that variables are free of the subjective judgement of observers. Objectivity exists where automated systems measure performance variables without human judgement involved in any part of the data collection. Where analysts record the decisions of others such as umpires and referees, the system is objective because the analyst is not making any judgements about performance. As has been explained in Chapter 2, other variables used in traditional notational analysis have varying degrees of objectivity depending on how matter-of-fact or obvious they are. For example, in tennis it may be easier to distinguish a forehand from a backhand than distinguishing between a forced and an unforced error. Performance indicators must have an objective measurement process which helps ensure validity. If the value recorded for a performance variable depends on subjective observer judgement too much, it could render the variable invalid.

## Reliability

Reliability is the consistency with which a measurement process can be applied. In sports performance analysis, if a system can analyse a sports performance consistently then it is reliable. This requires the system to produce similar results for performance variables each time it is used to analyse the same performance. Reliability is important in scientific research where the conclusions of studies may be used by practitioners. It is, therefore, essential that any study reports any limits in the reliability of the data used. This is also true when sports performance analysis is used in a coaching context. High performing athletes and their coaches will be making important decisions about preparation for forthcoming competition based on analyses done of recent performances by themselves and forthcoming opponents. Therefore, the data used must be of a sufficiently high quality to help avoid poor decisions about preparation.

## Sources of inaccuracy

James *et al.* (2002) classified errors made during performance analysis as:

- Definitional errors
- Perceptual errors
- Data entry errors

A definitional error is where a system has been defined using vague terms leading to operators interpreting performances in different ways. Even when lengthy definitions of events are specified, two independent observers may have different images in their minds about what the wordings of those definitions mean in terms of visual information about animated behaviour.

A perceptual error is where an operator mistakenly classifies behaviour using the wrong event type. This could occur due to the subjective nature of classifying some events such as unforced errors and forced errors. Players also use disguise and deception to gain an advantage over opponents and this may also take analysts recording behaviour by surprise. The model human information processing system in Chapter 2 (Figure 2.6) shows further sources of inaccuracy such as reaction time and motor

# 180

delays. There may be occasions where players are mistaken for other players, especially in sports where players in a team wear the same kit. Players may be obscured by other players or obstacles in the line of view.

Data entry errors occur when the operator recognises a movement correctly but presses the wrong button on the system interface.

## Intra-operator agreement

Given that there are subjective processes during human observation in sports performance analysis, the level of reliability needs to be tested and reported. This can be done using intra-operator and/or inter-operator agreement studies. An intra-operator agreement study is where an operator looks at the same performance twice (or more) using the given system to check the consistency of the results. This requires the performance to be video recorded for the second observation which occurs at least a week after the first observation. The gap of a week between observations is to reduce the chance of the operator recalling specific data entry events and to reduce the chance of the operator being able to predict what the player is about to do during the second observation. The results of the two observations can be compared highlighting areas where the operator is consistent and inconsistent in observation.

## Inter-operator agreement

The problem with intra-operator agreement is that it does not demonstrate objectivity of a system. Intra-operator agreement can determine that a given operator can analyse performances consistently. However, the question remains as to whether any other operators would agree with this operator about the performance recorded. Inter-operator agreement demonstrates the level of consistency achieved by different operators using the same system. The operators apply the system to the same performance independently. This could be simultaneously during live observation of the performance or it could be at different times using a video recording of the performance.

One might expect a greater level of intra-operator reliability than inter-operator reliability and this is typically what occurs. However, there are occasions where we might find a higher level of inter-operator agreement than intra-operator agreement. Essentially one observer is agreeing with another person more than agreeing with him/herself. This has been seen in published research. For example, McLaughlin and O'Donoghue (2001) found a higher level of inter-operator agreement than intra-operator agreement for a time-motion analysis system.

### Reliability studies

We need to justify the number of performances used in a reliability study. The figure of 40 or more allows certain types of reliability statistics to be used. However, the amount of time involved might be excessive in relation to the use of the system. If the system is going to be used to assess hundreds of performances over many seasons, a multiple performance reliability study may be justified. Where the system is to be used in a research project of 10 to 20 performances, a 40 performance reliability study is disproportionate compared to the effort involved in the main research. Therefore, single performance reliability studies are often used in sports performance analysis.

Reliability studies can also be classified by whether they investigate the reliability of the input data or the output variables that are produced. There is a case for saying that each performance indicator or output variable produced by a system must be tested for reliability. However, this may be very complex if there are many possible combinations of factors. For example, in the tennis serve system described in Chapter 6, there are 72 frequencies that can be tallied when we consider every combination of service court, first or second serve, area of the service court served to, type of serve and outcome. Indeed there may be word limits on scientific reports meaning that we would not be able to report the reliability of all potential system outputs. An alternative approach is to demonstrate the reliability of the input data that has been recorded and then use an inductive reasoning argument that reliable input data can lead to reliable outputs being derived from the input data.

### Relationship between objectivity, reliability and validity

The measurement concepts of objectivity, reliability and validity are related. Variables that are well defined are better understood by those

# 182

collecting the data used to create those variables. This can improve the consistency with which data are collected by different operators. The variable does need to be relevant and important to be valid and if it is not relevant and valid then the most detailed definitions and skilled data collection will not make it valid. However, an important and relevant concept does need to be measured reliably, otherwise its validity will be compromised. Validity is concerned with the extent to which a variable measures the concept it is intended to measure. If this is not done consistently, then measurement error can lead to values that are not realistic for individual performances.

Objectivity does not necessarily guarantee reliability. If we used a speed threshold such as 4m.s$^{-1}$ to distinguish jogging and running, we may have a precise definition, but it is not possible for human observers to recognise accurately the point in time when an accelerating or decelerating player reaches a speed of 4m.s$^{-1}$. If time-motion data have been measured automatically, for example using accelerometers or GPS devices, speed thresholds may be recognised more accurately but there may still be errors arising from the instruments used. The equipment would need to be tested to provide some understanding of such measurement issues.

There may also be occasions where objectivity may be at the expense of validity. For example, automatic player tracking systems may not distinguish between forward, backwards and sideways movement by the player. This can lead to an underestimation of the volume of high intensity activity that is performed because high intensity activity performed while moving backwards, sideways or even on-the-spot at speeds at less than 4m.s$^{-1}$ is classified as low intensity. For example, Redwood-Brown *et al.* (2009) found that English FA Premier League soccer players moved at speeds of 4m.s$^{-1}$ or faster for about 7 per cent of match time on average. The percentage of time spent performing high intensity activity by English FA Premier League soccer players is estimated to be between 10–11 per cent when using subjective judgement supported by general guidelines for what counts as high intensity activity (O'Donoghue *et al.*, 2005b). Another problem with using exact speed thresholds to distinguish movements such as jogging and running is that the speeds at which these movements are performed by the same players can overlap (Siegle and Lames, 2010).

## Computerised scoring in amateur boxing

The computerised scoring system that has been used in amateur boxing is an interesting example of measurement issues in sport. The computerised system for amateur boxing involves five judges who operate equipment allowing them to record the scoring punches they perceive to be made by the boxers wearing red and blue kit. A scoring punch is recorded if three or more of the five judges press a button of the same colour within 1s. This is essentially a judging application of performance analysis; the judges are observing and analysing the performance.

It can be claimed that the system is objective because there are criteria to be used by judges to recognise scoring punches. The punch should be made with the knuckle (white) part of the glove, to the front of the head or torso with the weight of the shoulder behind the punch. As with any guidelines given to human operators of performance analysis systems, there is some room for individual judge interpretation of the guidelines limiting inter-judge agreement.

Whether the system is valid is a matter of debate. A challenge to the validity of the system is that it counts the number of scoring punches made by each boxer without any distinction being made between punches of different qualities. The system makes no distinction between occasions where three, four or all five of the judges pressed a button of a given colour within 1s. However, in any sport the competitors try to maximise their chances of winning within the rules that are being applied. This might have changed the nature of amateur boxing as boxers will be aware that they can only score a maximum of one point per second. If a boxer were to use a rapid combination of punches and be hit by a single jab from the opponent, each boxer might score a single point from the exchange. Therefore, the use of combinations might be considered ineffective under the computerised scoring system.

Another way of looking at validity is whether the computerised scoring system produces a score that reflects the actual number of scoring punches made by each boxer during a bout. This would involve a detailed post-match video analysis to identify the correct number of scoring punches made. The score produced by the computerised scoring system would then be validated against this. The scores produced by the computerised scoring system typically underestimate the actual number of punches made that satisfy the criteria for a scoring punch (Coalter *et*

184

*al.*, 1998). This is because there may be occasions where more than one scoring punch is made in a second or because fewer than three judges press the correct button within 1s when a valid punch is made. This disagreement between individual judges is due to limited reliability.

The limited reliability is caused by perceptual and data entry errors. Judges may disagree about whether a punch satisfied the guidelines for a scoring punch. A judge may delay in pressing the appropriate button when a punch is made to the extent that the button press is not within the same one-second period as other judges recording the punch. There may be data entry errors where a judge presses the wrong button. Where delays in button pressing activity or pressing the incorrect button occur where two other judges have pressed a given button within a one-second period, the error will cost a boxer a point.

A system can actually be reliable without being accurate or valid if it produces a consistent wrong answer! Indeed, we could have a situation where all five judges press the red button more than the blue button but the boxer in blue is awarded more scoring punches by the computerised scoring system. This is because there may be more occasions where three or more judges press the blue button within one second than the red button despite the fact that all five judges press the red button more often than the blue button. So in considering the reliability of the judges' scores we need to be mindful that reliability is not the only important measurement issue. The reliability of the judging activity can be evaluated by comparing the frequencies of red and blue button presses between each pair of judges. The frequency data conceal the number of occasions where the two judges press the same button at the same time. Therefore, a better reliability study could analyse the occasions where the button pressing activity of a pair of judges agree and disagree. There are statistical techniques such as coefficient of variation and intra-class correlation coefficient that can measure the level of agreement between all five judges which could be used here.

## RELIABILITY STATISTICS FOR CATEGORICAL VARIABLES

### Categorical variables

A categorical variable is one that has a finite number of named values. For example, the variable Service Type may have the values Flat Serve,

Kick Serve and Slice Serve. There are two types of categorical variables; nominal variables and ordinal variables. Service Type is a nominal variable because the types of serve have no order; they are just different values that the variable could take. An ordinal variable, on the other hand, has a finite number of values that have an order whereby some values are considered greater than others. For example, we may have a variable outcome that represents the outcome of a possession in soccer. The value of this variable could be Goal, Shot on target, Shot off target, Entered the attacking third or Unsuccessful. These values have been expressed here in descending order of achievement in that Goal is a more preferable outcome to a Shot on target which is a more preferable outcome to a Shot off target, and so on. In this section of the chapter, the tennis serve example covered in Chapters 6 and 8 is used to show the calculation of percentage error (Hughes *et al.*, 2004) and kappa (Cohen, 1960). The tennis example includes five variables of interest:

- The court that was served to (deuce or advantage).
- The service (1st or 2nd).
- The type of serve (Flat, Kick or Slice).
- The area of the service court served to (Left, Middle or Right).
- The outcome of the point (Won or Lost by the server).

In the exercises done in Chapter 6 there were 23 points to the deuce court and 27 to the advantage court. This is actually not possible as all games start with the server serving to the deuce court and finish with the server serving to either the deuce or the advantage court. Therefore, the number of points where the server serves to the advantage court cannot exceed the number served to the deuce court. What has happened is that the double faults were not recorded because the ball did not land in the left, middle or right of the target service box on either the first or second serve. There are actually six double faults served as shown by the blank rows in Table 9.1. Therefore we have 56 points instead of 50. Table 9.1 shows the data entered for these 56 points by two independent observers. The reliability analysis described in this chapter simply considers the 50 points where a serve was in. We would not actually be aware of what each observer recorded for individual points if we used the tally system (frequency table) described in Chapter 6. However, the computerised version described in Chapter 8 does provide such an Event List as well as the summary frequencies.

# 186

## Percentage error

Given two values for the frequency of an event recorded by independent observers, V1 and V2, Hughes *et al.* (2004) defined percentage error as shown in equation (9.1).

$$\%\text{Error} = 100 \times |\,V1 - V2\,|/((V1+V2)/2) \qquad (9.1)$$

Here, $|V1 - V2|$ is the magnitude of the error. In other words, we determine the difference between the two values but do not include the sign (+ or −) of the difference. We cannot assume that it is the first or second observer who has recorded the correct frequency. Indeed they might both have recorded the incorrect frequency for the given event. Therefore, the difference in their values is expressed as a percentage of the mean of their two values. For example, if one observer recorded 19 and the other recorded 21, the difference of 2 would be 10 per cent of the mean of their two values (20). Thus the percentage effort is 10 per cent where one observer recorded 19 and the other records 21.

As Table 9.1 shows, the only errors that occurred were in the recording of serve type and area served to. The percentage errors for these are summarised in Table 9.2. Remember that percentage error is being calculated from frequencies tallied and typically analysts would not have a list of points, such as Table 9.1, available to them. Note that Table 9.2 does not show the difference, absolute difference or mean value between the two observers. Once we have stated that we are using percentage error (Hughes *et al.*, 2004), the method used to evaluate percentage error is known and the detail of percentage error can be looked up from the original source by those unfamiliar with it. As an exercise, calculate the percentage error for each serve type and area served to and see if you agree with the values in Table 9.2. We would probably not include Serve, Court and Outcome in such a Table as we could simply state in a sentence that there were no disagreements in the frequencies of these variables. One thing we can observe from Table 9.2 is that a single disagreement can result in two percentage error values being greater than 0.0 per cent. For example, if Observer 1 judges a serve to be a flat serve and Observer 2 observes it to be a kick serve, then their frequencies for flat and kick serves will disagree. Another thing we can observe from Table 9.2 is that single disagreements result in greater percentage errors with low frequencies than with higher frequencies. For example, the difference of one is a 4.7

Table 9.1 Data entered for 56 tennis points

| Game | Point | Observer 1 | | | | | Observer 2 | | | | | Error |
|---|---|---|---|---|---|---|---|---|---|---|---|---|
| | | COURT | SERVE | TYPE | AREA | OUTCOME | COURT | SERVE | TYPE | AREA | OUTCOME | |
| 1 | 1 | Deuce | 1 | Flat | Left | Won | Deuce | 1 | Kick | Left | Won | Yes |
| 1 | 2 | Adv | 1 | Flat | Right | Won | Adv | 1 | Flat | Right | Won | |
| 1 | 3 | Deuce | | | | | Deuce | | | | | |
| 1 | 4 | Adv | 2 | Slice | Middle | Lost | Adv | 2 | Slice | Middle | Lost | |
| 1 | 5 | Deuce | 1 | Slice | Left | Won | Deuce | 1 | Slice | Left | Won | |
| 1 | 6 | Adv | 1 | Flat | Left | Won | Adv | 1 | Flat | Left | Won | |
| 2 | 1 | Deuce | 2 | Slice | Middle | Lost | Deuce | 2 | Slice | Middle | Lost | |
| 2 | 2 | Adv | 1 | Slice | Left | Won | Adv | 1 | Slice | Left | Won | |
| 2 | 3 | Deuce | | | | | Deuce | | | | | |
| 2 | 4 | Adv | 2 | Slice | Middle | Lost | Adv | 2 | Slice | Middle | Lost | |
| 2 | 5 | Deuce | 1 | Slice | Left | Lost | Deuce | 1 | Slice | Left | Lost | |
| 3 | 1 | Deuce | 1 | Slice | Middle | Won | Deuce | 1 | Slice | Middle | Won | |
| 3 | 2 | Adv | 1 | Flat | Right | Won | Adv | 1 | Flat | Right | Won | |
| 3 | 3 | Deuce | 1 | Kick | Left | Won | Deuce | 1 | Flat | Left | Won | Yes |
| 3 | 4 | Adv | 1 | Flat | Left | Won | Adv | 1 | Flat | Left | Won | |
| 4 | 1 | Deuce | 2 | Kick | Right | Won | Deuce | 2 | Kick | Middle | Won | Yes |
| 4 | 2 | Adv | 2 | Flat | Middle | Won | Adv | 2 | Flat | Middle | Won | |
| 4 | 3 | Deuce | 2 | Kick | Middle | Lost | Deuce | 2 | Kick | Middle | Lost | |
| 4 | 4 | Adv | 1 | Flat | Middle | Lost | Adv | 1 | Flat | Left | Lost | Yes |
| 4 | 5 | Deuce | 1 | Flat | Right | Won | Deuce | 1 | Flat | Right | Won | |
| 4 | 6 | Adv | 2 | Flat | Middle | Won | Adv | 2 | Kick | Middle | Won | Yes |
| 5 | 1 | Deuce | 2 | Flat | Middle | Lost | Deuce | 2 | Flat | Middle | Lost | |
| 5 | 2 | Adv | 2 | Flat | Left | Won | Adv | 2 | Flat | Left | Won | |
| 5 | 3 | Deuce | | | | | Deuce | | | | | |
| 5 | 4 | Adv | 1 | Slice | Left | Lost | Adv | 1 | Slice | Left | Lost | |
| 5 | 5 | Deuce | 1 | Kick | Left | Lost | Deuce | 1 | Kick | Left | Lost | |
| 6 | 1 | Deuce | 2 | Slice | Middle | Won | Deuce | 2 | Slice | Middle | Won | |
| 6 | 2 | Adv | 2 | Flat | Middle | Lost | Adv | 2 | Flat | Middle | Lost | |

Table 9.1 continued

| Game | Point | Observer 1 | | | | | Observer 2 | | | | | |
|---|---|---|---|---|---|---|---|---|---|---|---|---|
| | | COURT | SERVE | TYPE | AREA | OUTCOME | COURT | SERVE | TYPE | AREA | OUTCOME | Error |
| 6 | 3 | Deuce | 1 | Flat | Middle | Won | Deuce | 1 | Flat | Right | Won | Yes |
| 6 | 4 | Adv | 2 | Slice | Middle | Lost | Adv | 2 | Slice | Middle | Lost | |
| 6 | 5 | Deuce | 2 | Slice | Left | Won | Deuce | 2 | Slice | Left | Won | |
| 6 | 6 | Adv | 1 | Slice | Left | Won | Adv | 1 | Slice | Left | Won | |
| 7 | 1 | Deuce | | | | | Deuce | | | | | |
| 7 | 2 | Adv | 1 | Slice | Right | Won | Adv | 1 | Slice | Middle | Won | Yes |
| 7 | 3 | Deuce | 1 | Flat | Left | Won | Deuce | 1 | Flat | Left | Won | |
| 7 | 4 | Adv | 1 | Slice | Left | Lost | Adv | 1 | Slice | Left | Lost | |
| 7 | 5 | Deuce | | | | | Deuce | | | | | |
| 7 | 6 | Adv | 1 | Kick | Right | Won | Adv | 1 | Flat | Right | Won | Yes |
| 7 | 7 | Deuce | 1 | Slice | Right | Won | Deuce | 1 | Slice | Right | Won | |
| 7 | 8 | Adv | 1 | Flat | Left | Won | Adv | 1 | Flat | Left | Won | |
| 8 | 1 | Deuce | 2 | Flat | Middle | Won | Deuce | 2 | Flat | Middle | Won | |
| 8 | 2 | Adv | 1 | Kick | Right | Lost | Adv | 1 | Kick | Right | Lost | |
| 8 | 3 | Deuce | 2 | Slice | Middle | Won | Deuce | 2 | Slice | Middle | Won | |
| 8 | 4 | Adv | 1 | Flat | Left | Lost | Adv | 1 | Kick | Left | Lost | Yes |
| 8 | 5 | Deuce | 2 | Kick | Middle | Won | Deuce | 2 | Kick | Middle | Won | |
| 8 | 6 | Adv | 1 | Flat | Left | Lost | Adv | 1 | Flat | Left | Lost | |
| 8 | 7 | Deuce | 2 | Flat | Middle | Lost | Deuce | 2 | Flat | Middle | Lost | |
| 8 | 8 | Adv | 1 | Kick | Left | Won | Adv | 1 | Flat | Left | Won | Yes |
| 8 | 9 | Deuce | 2 | Slice | Left | Lost | Deuce | 2 | Slice | Left | Lost | |
| 8 | 10 | Adv | 1 | Slice | Left | Won | Adv | 1 | Slice | Left | Won | |
| 8 | 11 | Deuce | | | | | Deuce | | | | | |
| 8 | 12 | Adv | 2 | Slice | Middle | Won | Adv | 2 | Slice | Middle | Won | |
| 8 | 13 | Deuce | 1 | Flat | Right | Won | Deuce | 1 | Flat | Right | Won | |
| 8 | 14 | Adv | 1 | Flat | Right | Lost | Adv | 1 | Flat | Right | Lost | |
| 8 | 15 | Deuce | 1 | Flat | Right | Won | Deuce | 1 | Kick | Right | Won | Yes |
| 8 | 16 | Adv | 2 | Kick | Middle | Won | Adv | 2 | Kick | Middle | Won | |

Table 9.2 Percentage error of frequencies for different variables

| Variable | Observer 1 | Observer 2 | % Error |
|---|---|---|---|
| *Serve* | | | |
| 1st | 30 | 30 | 0.0 |
| 2nd | 20 | 20 | 0.0 |
| *Court* | | | |
| Deuce | 23 | 23 | 0.0 |
| Adv | 27 | 27 | 0.0 |
| *Type* | | | |
| Flat | 22 | 21 | 4.7 |
| Kick | 9 | 10 | 10.5 |
| Slice | 19 | 19 | 0.0 |
| *Area* | | | |
| Left | 20 | 21 | 4.9 |
| Middle | 19 | 19 | 0.0 |
| Right | 11 | 10 | 9.5 |
| *Outcome* | | | |
| Won | 32 | 32 | 0.0 |
| Lost | 18 | 18 | 0.0 |

per cent error for a flat serve but a 10.5 per cent error for the kick serve. If we had a single disagreement whereby one observer recorded a frequency of one for an event and the other recorded a frequency of zero, the percentage error would be calculated as 200 per cent which looks really serious, but it is just one error. Therefore, students need to step back and look at whole variables such as serve type rather than each individual serve type value when evaluating reliability data. Both observers are broadly agreeing that the frequencies of flat and slice serves are similar while fewer kick serves are played. Is this level of agreement between the operators good enough? Well, it depends on what the system is being used for. In some cases the minor difference in frequency distributions may be entirely acceptable but in other situations it may be problematic. Therefore, we need to consider reliability and error levels in relation to the analytical goals of the analysis. Do the levels of reliability for serve type and area served to differ between deuce and advantage courts, between first and second serve points or indeed between different combinations of serve and court served to? This level of detail could be determined from the frequency table used in Chapter 6. There are 72

# 190

different raw frequencies when we consider combinations of all five variables. There are additional higher order frequencies that can be derived when we consider two, three or four variables together. However, the frequencies of points in individual cells may be very low; for example in Figure 6.6 the maximum frequency is 4. This could lead to high percentage error values for single errors and a cumbersome analysis of system reliability being presented. Therefore, any combinations of variables for which reliability statistics are to be calculated need to be justified by their importance in decision making when the system is being used.

## Kappa

There are no summary frequencies in Table 9.2 that differ by more than 1 between the two observers for any variable. However, these summary frequencies may conceal errors that have cancelled each other out. Consider Table 9.3 which can be derived from the data in Table 9.1 using a pivot table in Excel. Consider, in particular, the frequencies recorded for the kick serve; 9 by Observer 1 and 10 by Observer 2. There may only be a difference of 1 between these two frequencies but there were actually only six points where both observers agreed that the serve was a kick serve. Where we have an Event List from a computerised system such as the tennis system described in Chapter 8, or from a manual sequential system, we can produce a cross-tabulation of frequencies such as that shown in Table 9.3. This allows the number of points where the observers agreed to be determined. For example, there are 43 points where the observers agree on type of serve and 46 points where they agree on the area served to. These are the sum of the frequencies on the top-left to bottom-right diagonals of Tables 9.3(a) and (b) respectively. When these are divided by the total number of points (50), we get $P_0$ which is the proportion of points where the observers agree. This is 0.86 for type of serve ( $(18 + 6 + 19)/50 = 43/50 = 0.86$ ) and 0.92 for area served to ( $(20 + 17 + 9)/50 = 46/50 = 0.92$ ).

The proportion of agreed events could be expressed as a percentage of agreed events by simply multiplying by 100. Therefore, the observers agree on the type of serve for 86 per cent of points and they agree on the area served to for 92 per cent of points. However, the proportion of agreed events, $P_0$, and the corresponding percentage do not address the proportion of events we would expect to be agreed by chance. Imagine if

Observer 2 had decided to guess the type of serve used in each point, but using the proportions 21 flat serves, 10 kick serves and 19 slice serves for 50 points. This means that for each point there is a 21/50 = 0.42 chance that Observer 2 will guess that the serve is a flat serve. This does not matter when Observer 1 records a kick or a slice serve. However, on each of the 22 occasions where Observer 1 records a flat serve, there is a 0.42 chance of Observer 2 agreeing just by guessing! This amounts to 22 × (21/50) = 9.24 agreements that the serve is a flat serve by guessing. Similarly, we would expect 9 × (10/50) = 1.80 agreements by guessing that the serve is a kick serve and 19 × (19/50) = 7.22 agreements by guessing that the serve is a slice serve. When the expected frequencies for the observers agreeing by guessing are added together, we get a sum of 18.26 agreements for serve type that we would expect to agree by guessing. This gives an expected proportion of points where serve could be agreed by guessing of 18.26/50 = 0.365.

The kappa statistic, $\kappa$, adjusts the proportion of agreements, $P_0$, by the proportion of occasions where we would be expected to agree by guessing, $P_C$. The best way to think about the adjustment is to consider $P_0$ to be itself divided by one. Now if we subtract $P_C$ away from the top and bottom of this division, we get kappa as shown in equation (9.2). Therefore, the kappa value for type of point, $\kappa = (0.86 - 0.365)/(1 - 0.365)$ = 0.780. Table 9.3(b) shows the $P_0$, $P_C$ and $\kappa$ values for area served to. See if you can make these calculations using the cross-tabulated frequencies and agree with the values given for $P_0$, $P_C$ and $\kappa$.

$$\kappa = (P_0 - P_C)/(1 - P_C) \tag{9.2}$$

Table 9.3 Cross-tabulation of frequency of events recorded by two independent observers (Observer 1 and Observer 2)

| (a) Type of serve | | | | | (b) Area served to | | | | |
|---|---|---|---|---|---|---|---|---|---|
| Observer 1 | Observer 2 | | | | Observer 1 | Observer 2 | | | |
| | Flat | Kick | Slice | Total | | Left | Mid | Right | Total |
| Flat | 18 | 4 | 0 | 22 | Left | 20 | 0 | 0 | 20 |
| Kick | 3 | 6 | 0 | 9 | Mid | 1 | 17 | 1 | 19 |
| Slice | 0 | 0 | 19 | 19 | Right | 0 | 2 | 9 | 11 |
| Total | 21 | 10 | 19 | 50 | Total | 21 | 19 | 10 | 50 |
| $P_0$ | 0.860 | | | | $P_0$ | 0.920 | | | |
| $P_C$ | 0.365 | | | | $P_C$ | 0.356 | | | |
| $\kappa$ | 0.789 | | | | $\kappa$ | 0.876 | | | |

## Interpretation of kappa

Altman (1991: 404) classified kappa values as very good, good, moderate, fair or poor in an applied medical science example. The strength of agreement between observations is interpreted as follows:

$0.8 \leq \kappa \leq 1.0$: Very good
$0.6 \leq \kappa < 0.8$: Good
$0.4 \leq \kappa < 0.6$: Moderate
$0.2 \leq \kappa < 0.4$: Fair
$0.0 \leq \kappa < 0.2$: Poor
$-1.0 \leq \kappa < 0.0$: Very poor

Negative values occur where the level of agreement is lower than would be expected by guessing. Kappa values less than 0.0 should be classified as very poor.

## Matching events

The tennis example is relatively straightforward because we at least know that there are 50 points where a serve was played in. The other example used in Chapters 6 and 8 was the analysis of possessions in soccer. It is possible that two independent observers might not even agree on the number of possessions that have occurred in a game. It is necessary to identify event records in one observer's Event List that correspond to event records in the other observer's Event List. This matching process is typically manual, even if the data have been collected using a computerised system. Basically, an analyst needs to place corresponding Event Lists side by side in Excel and move many records for each observer so that any row in the spreadsheet only contains information for a single event. The single event in a given row of the spreadsheet might have been recorded by one or both of the observers.

There are many different reasons why events may be recorded by one observer but not the other. There may be occasions where a ball was briefly touched by a player of one team before being lost again to the opposition. Table 9.4 shows an example of this derived from the example in Chapter 6 (Figure 6.9). Recall that the two teams are referred to as 'Us' and 'Them'. Here, Observer 2 has analysed the same match section

**Table 9.4** A section of match data where two observers disagree on the number of possessions that have occurred

| Observer 1 | | | | | Observer 2 | | | | |
|---|---|---|---|---|---|---|---|---|---|
| Time | Team | Posses-sion | Area | Outcome | Time | Team | Posses-sion | Area | Outcome |
| 00:00 | Us | KO | CM | | 00:00 | Us | KO | CM | |
| 00:15 | Them | IN | CD | | 00:15 | Them | IN | CD | |
| 00:22 | Us | TK | RM | Shot | 00:22 | Us | TK | RM | Shot |
| | | | | | 00:28 | Them | IN | CM | |
| | | | | | 00:29 | Us | IM | CM | |
| 00:34 | Them | IN | CD | Score | 00:34 | Them | IN | CD | Score |
| 00:48 | Us | KO | CM | | 00:48 | Us | KO | CM | |

but has added a possession for 'Them' at 28s into the match Event List which has effectively split the possession recorded by Observer 1 at 22s into two because the new possession occurred in the middle of it. Therefore, by the time the match reaches 48s, Observer 2 has already recorded two more possessions than Observer 1. There may also be occasions where Observer 1 records possessions that are not recorded by Observer 2. These mismatches are not a problem in a frequency table where percentage errors can be calculated for the variables. However, with a sequential system, these mismatches necessitate the need for additional 'none' values for each variable. For example, there are seven possession types but, for the purpose of reliability, we also need to represent where no possession has been recorded. Consider Table 9.5 which cross-tabulates frequencies for possession types recorded by the two observers. There are eight occasions where Observer 1 has recorded a possession but Observer 2 has not and 10 occasions where Observer 2 has recorded a possession but Observer 1 has not. This means that rather than there being 168 possessions, there are only 150 possessions that have been agreed to have occurred by the two observers and in some of these cases they do not agree on the type of possession. We do not actually know the real number of possessions. We only know that Observer 1 has recorded 158 possessions and Observer 2 has recorded 160. We cannot exclude the 18 possession records that have only been identified by a single observer because this would conceal genuine disagreements between the observers. The fact that we cannot have a frequency in the bottom right-hand cell (where neither observer recorded an event) makes this a harsh calculation of kappa. We can have an agreement by chance

# 194

Table 9.5 Cross-tabulation of possession types including occasions where only one observer recorded a possession

| Observer 1 | Observer 2 | | | | | | | | |
| --- | --- | --- | --- | --- | --- | --- | --- | --- | --- |
| | Kick off | Tackle | Inter-ception | Throw in | Corner kick | Goal kick | Free | None | Total |
| Kick off | 4 | | | | | | | | 4 |
| Tackle | | 16 | 2 | | | | | 1 | 19 |
| Interception | | 1 | 41 | | | | | 7 | 49 |
| Throw in | | | | 26 | | | | | 26 |
| Corner | | | | | 11 | | | | 11 |
| Goal kick | | | | | | 13 | 1 | | 14 |
| Free kick | | | | | | | 35 | | 35 |
| None | | 2 | 8 | | | | | | 10 |
| Total | 4 | 19 | 51 | 26 | 11 | 13 | 36 | 8 | 168 |

for 'none' but we cannot have any agreement recorded for 'none'. In this particular example, $P_0$ is 0.869, $P_C$ is 0.184 so kappa is 0.840.

One of the issues with this use of kappa is that it determines the reliability of the input data on a variable by variable basis. For example in the tennis system, we would have kappa values for service court, service (first or second), type of serve, area served to and point outcome. We may prefer to produce reliability statistics for the system output variables such as the frequency of first serve points or the percentage of first serve points that are won by the server. This would require us to use a reliability statistic such as percentage error rather than kappa.

## RELIABILITY IN TIME-MOTION ANALYSIS

### Time-motion analysis

In Chapter 1, work-rate analysis was one of two main purposes of sports performance analysis that were introduced. Work-rate analysis is a type of time-motion analysis with other types of time-motion analysis including the analysis of rally and rest times in racket sports. Time-motion analysis can be done using subjective classification of movement by trained observers operating time-motion systems or more objectively using semi-automatic player tracking systems as discussed in Chapter 2. In time-motion analysis we have a nominal variable such as movement type which has a set of nominal values such as the seven suggested by Huey *et al.* (2001):

- Stationary – this included standing, sitting, stretching or lying in a prone position.
- Walking – walking forwards.
- Backing – walking in a backwards or sideways direction.
- Jogging – slow running movement without obvious effort or acceleration.
- Running – running with obvious effort through to all out sprinting.
- Shuffling – shuffling backwards or sideways or on-the-spot shuffling movement with the feet.
- Game related activity – ball contact during ball-in-play time or challenging for the ball.

These definitions offer some guidance to operators. However, there is still considerable subjective observer judgement during data gathering. Consider the definition of jogging. The operator needs to make a judgement about effort. Indeed, there will be some effort as the player will be using energy when jogging at any speed. So the operator needs to be aware that the words 'obvious effort' really means high intensity effort when we are considering running. Walking, jogging and shuffling are defined recursively using the words walking, jogging and running respectively. The distinction between walking and jogging could use the regulations applied in race walking that at least one foot has to be in contact with the ground all the time when walking. Once the movement involves any periods, however short, where both feet are off the ground, the movement is no longer walking. There is still a great deal of scope for different interpretations of movement. Those who conduct such analyses face an impossible task if they aim to produce a set of definitions that can be used identically by any trained human operators. It is, therefore, common to provide guidance to assist operators up to the point where further detail would provide negligible improvement to reliability or even be counter-productive.

These seven nominal values are not merely counted in time-motion analysis but they are also timed. For example, an athlete might have jogged 15 times with the total amount of time spent jogging being 120s. This allows us to also determine that the mean duration of an instance of jogging was 8s. In Chapter 1, Tables 1.3 and 1.4 show the frequency,

# 196

mean duration and percentage observation time for different movement types. In writing the current chapter, the author and a colleague independently analysed a 97-minute video recording that followed a single professional football player for an entire English FA Premier League match. This was done using a computerised time-motion analysis system that was tailored to include the seven movements.

The two data sets were compared by a reliability assessment routine that implemented a timed version of kappa (O'Donoghue, 2005b). Rather than determining the frequency of occasions where two observers agree on some movement type, the timed versions of kappa determines the amount of time (in s) where the two observers agree. Table 9.6 shows the amount of time where the two observers recorded different activities. Because the start and end times of movements will often be recorded at slightly different times by the two observers, there will be disagreements even when they agree on the movements being performed. For example, when both observers record jogging and then running, but one observer records the start of the run 0.2s after the other observer. This will lead to a 0.2s of observation time where one observer recorded jogging and the other recorded running. In Table 9.6, the total amount of time where the two observers agreed on the movement performed was 4362.73s (72 mins 42.73s) out of the total observation time of 5821.50s (97 mins 1.50s). A large proportion of this agreed time is where both observers agreed that the player was stationary, walking, backing or jogging which were performed for a greater percentage of match time than other activities. The amount of time where the observers agreed the player was shuffling

Table 9.6 Time recorded (s) for soccer player movement by two independent observers using a seven-movement classification scheme

| Observer 1 | Observer 2 | | | | | | | |
| | Stationary | Walking | Backing | Jogging | Running | Shuffling | Game rel | Total |
| --- | --- | --- | --- | --- | --- | --- | --- | --- |
| Stationary | 581.19 | 42.09 | 18.87 | 1.70 | 4.55 | 5.23 | 3.23 | 656.86 |
| Walking | 214.27 | 2,705.2 | 132.63 | 130.26 | 25.51 | 45.61 | 14.89 | 3,268.37 |
| Backing | 89.34 | 109.43 | 436.72 | 8.14 | 3.94 | 24.10 | 2.82 | 674.49 |
| Jogging | 20.66 | 148.90 | 22.51 | 474.03 | 105.07 | 94.29 | 30.04 | 895.50 |
| Running | 2.70 | 8.81 | 0.66 | 9.53 | 66.93 | 8.79 | 12.91 | 110.33 |
| Shuffling | 8.23 | 16.13 | 15.14 | 19.21 | 16.15 | 54.57 | 15.91 | 145.34 |
| Game rel | 2.08 | 3.51 | 1.97 | 5.32 | 9.58 | 4.06 | 44.09 | 70.61 |
| Total | 918.47 | 3,034.07 | 628.50 | 648.19 | 231.73 | 236.65 | 123.89 | 5,821.50 |

is less than 50 per cent of the time that either observer recorded shuffling. Once we have determined the timings shown in Table 9.6, the calculation of kappa is identical to the way it is used with frequency data. $P_0$ is 0.749, $P_C$ is 0.342 and, therefore, kappa is 0.619 indicating a good strength of agreement according to Altman's (1991) classification.

Interestingly, trying to improve reliability by combining different types of work (running, shuffling and game related activity) into a single 'work' activity and doing the same with rest activities reduces the kappa values from 0.619 to 0.469 which represents a moderate strength of agreement. The amount of time where each observer recorded 'rest' and 'work' is shown in Table 9.7. What has happened is that because soccer players spend about 90 per cent of match time in rest activity, there is a very high probability of agreeing by chance. Indeed if Observer 1 were to just record rest activities and nothing else, this would agree with Observer 2 for 94.4 per cent of observation time. This is why we use kappa rather than just $P_0$. If Observer 1 had only recorded 'rest' activities in this case, the kappa value would actually be 0.0. This is because $P_0$ and $P_C$ would be identical. Students are encouraged to set up a 2 × 2 table to test what kappa is evaluated to in such a situation. Given the data shown in Table 9.7, the $P_C$ value of 0.854 adjusts the $P_0$ value (0.922) to give the kappa value of 0.469.

The reliability of time-motion analysis could be improved by simply using a two-movement classification scheme (work and rest) where these two-movement types are entered directly rather than being determined from seven-movement classification data. Table 9.8 shows the amount of time recorded for rest and work by the two independent observers for the English FA Premier League player when using the two-movement classification scheme. $P_0$ is 0.965, $P_C$ is 0.846 with kappa being 0.772 which is a good strength of agreement.

Table 9.7 Combining the different types of rest and combining the different types of work (values in s)

| Observer 1 | | Observer 2 | |
| | Rest | Work | Total |
| --- | --- | --- | --- |
| Rest | 5,135.94 | 359.28 | 5,495.22 |
| Work | 93.29 | 232.99 | 326.28 |
| Total | 5,229.23 | 592.27 | 5,821.50 |

# 198

Table 9.8 Time recorded (s) for soccer player movement by two independent observers using a two-movement classification scheme

| Observer 1 | Observer 2 | | |
| | Rest | Work | Total |
| --- | --- | --- | --- |
| Rest | 5,214.93 | 68.20 | 5,283.13 |
| Work | 135.20 | 385.07 | 520.27 |
| Total | 5,350.13 | 453.27 | 5,803.40 |

## Operationalising low and moderate to high intensity activity

There may be situations in time-motion analysis or other purposes of sports performance analysis where precise operational definitions are possible. Imagine if a time-motion study simply wished to distinguish between low intensity activity (comprising of low intensity stationary movement and walking) and moderate to high intensity activity (comprising of jogging, running and sprinting for example). The system developers might decide to define low intensity movement as any movement where some part of the player's body is in contact with the ground for periods of 1s or longer. This could include lying in a prone position, single stepping and walking. The reason for specifying a minimum period of 1s or longer is that running does involve feet striking the ground. Therefore, we need to ensure that an operator is not classifying every foot strike of a run or sprint as low intensity activity just because the player's foot struck the ground. Some will argue that there is some high intensity activity that can be performed when at least one foot is on the ground for a period of over one second. Indeed, the winning time of 1 hour 18 minutes and 46s by China's Ding Chen 2012 Olympic 20km walk is equivalent to 6 minutes and 20s for each mile. I am sure many readers can run a mile in this time, but for many readers it is not a low intensity activity. Despite this limitation, the definition could potentially be applied by independent operators to produce consistent results for the analysis of the same performances. The idea is that the operators gather data based on the definition used to distinguish low intensity activity from moderate to high intensity activity without being influenced by their own common-sense subjective judgement of the intensity of the movement observed. There will still be sources of inaccuracy. For example, where a player rapidly starts running having been in a stationary position, one operator may react quicker to this than another operator.

There may be a situation where a player is jogging and momentarily slows to a walk and then starts jogging again. One operator may record the momentary walk as low intensity movement and the other operator might not be quick enough to react to it. It is also possible that such a momentary movement could be missed if an operator glanced down at their computer screen just to check the data entry was still functioning. Therefore, given such sources of inaccuracy even when we have precise operational definitions, it is necessary to do a reliability study of the method.

**Meaningful reliability assessment**

The classification scheme for kappa proposed by Altman (1991: 404) has been used in applied medical science research. However, it may not be suitable for time-motion analysis. Consider the binary movement classification (work and rest), example, results of which are summarised in Table 9.8. In this section of the chapter, we will use kappa as a measure of inter-operator agreement and deliberately introduce errors into synthetic data to look at different severities of error that could be made during data collection. Consider a 15-minute observation period (900s) where one observer records a 6s burst of high intensity activity starting every 25s. Therefore, there is 19s low intensity recovery between each 6-second burst with a total of 36 work bursts and 36 rest intervals being performed during the 15-minute observation period. Now imagine that a second observer records all of the odd six-second bursts of high intensity activity (first, third, fifth, ..., thirty-fifth) that were recorded by the first observer, but does not record the even bursts. Therefore, the second observer has recorded 18 busts of 6s with recoveries of 44s (19s + 6s + 19s) in between them. Figure 9.1 represents the work and rest periods recorded by the two observers.

In summary, the first observer has recorded work for 24 per cent of the observation with 36 bursts of work lasting 6s and 36 recoveries lasting 19s. The second observer has recorded work for 12 per cent of the observation period with 18 bursts of 6s and 18 recoveries of 44s. Is this a serious disagreement between the two observers or are they broadly agreeing that the activity is intermittent high intensity activity with repeated bursts of six seconds? In a situation like this, we need to forget about what the statisticians say about acceptable percentage error values

# 200

Observer 1

| 6s | 19s | 6s | 19s | 6s | 19s | 6s | 19s | | 6s | 19s | 6s | 19s |

Observer 2

| 6s | 44s | 6s | 44s | | 6s | 44s |

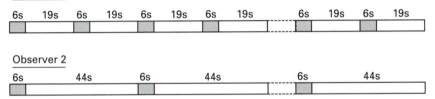

**Figure 9.1** An arbitrary situation where Observer 2 records half of the work periods recorded by Observer 1

and kappa values that indicate a good strength of inter-operator agreement. We need to consider the nature of sports performance and whether the different movement patterns recorded are similar enough or unacceptably different. The first place the author looked in this situation was the physiology laboratory experiment of Hughes *et al.* (2005) where heart rate, blood lactate and power output were measured when participants did 10 × 6s bursts with varying recoveries. There were three conditions; six-second bursts every 25s, six-second bursts every 45s and six-second bursts every 55s. The study found no significant difference in responses to bursts performed every 45s and every 55s. However, when the six-second bursts were performed every 25s, there was a significantly higher heart rate response, significantly higher blood lactate measures taken and significantly lower power output during the latter repetitions compared to when the participants took 45s and 55s recovery between six-second bursts.

This laboratory study suggested that the energy systems utilised when 6s bursts are performed every 25s are different from when six-second bursts are performed every 50s (half way between two of Hughes *et al.*'s conditions). Therefore, the two observers have failed to record reliably; it is as if they are looking at two different types of intermittent high intensity activity. Table 9.9 shows the amount of observation time where the two observers agreed and disagreed. The two observers agreed on the activity for ($P_0$ =) 0.88 of the observation time. The probability of agreeing by guessing is ($P_C$ = ) 0.6976. The expected time they could be expected to agree on work by guessing was 108 × 216/900 = 25.92s. The expected time they could be expected to agree on rest by guessing was

Table 9.9 Synthetic reliability data for time motion analysis

| Observer 1 | | Observer 2 | |
| | Work | Rest | Total |
| --- | --- | --- | --- |
| Work | 18 × 6s = 108s | 18 × 6s = 108s | 216s |
| Rest | 0s | 36 × 19s = 684s | 684s |
| Total | 108s | 792s | 900s |

$792 \times 684/900 = 601.92s$. When the total time they could be expected to agree of 627.84s is divided by the observation time of 900s we get the figure of 0.6976 for $P_C$. Kappa, $\kappa = (P_0 - P_C)/(1 - P_C) = (0.88 - 0.6976)/(1 - 0.6976) = 0.6032$ which is a good strength of agreement according to Altman (1991: 404). This is quite alarming when we consider that the observers would be concluding different types of intermittent high intensity activity being performed. Essentially, Altman's evaluation scheme for kappa was developed for use in applied medical research. He used an example of xerograms being interpreted by different radiologists. Time-motion data is a different application area and we are looking at a volume of agreed time during corresponding observations of a player, rather than frequencies of agreements for discrete assessments. This suggests that a kappa value of 0.6 is below what is an acceptable level of agreement for the binary work-rate analysis system.

We also need to consider that in a realistic example, it would be most unlikely that all bursts would be 6s and even if they were, those that were agreed might have a short period at the beginning and end that differed due to differing start times and end times for bursts being recorded by the two observers. The differences in start times and the differences in end times could result from observer fatigue, motor delays during data entry as well as differing perceptions of when a work (or rest) period started (or ended). This would lower the kappa value to around 0.537. This happens if the work-work agreement is reduced to 18 × 5.5s with 0.5s on either side of the 5.5s periods being the work-rest and rest-work disagreements. This is illustrated in Figure 9.2. Table 9.10 shows the impact these minor differences in start times and end times have on the amount of time the observers agree on work and rest.

If we consider three broad conclusions from a reliability study as being good, acceptable and poor agreement, then what we need to determine

# 202

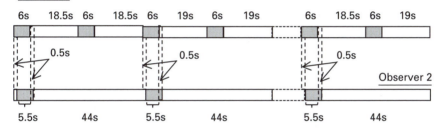

**Figure 9.2** An arbitrary situation where Observer 2 records half of the work periods recorded by Observer 1. In this example, the start and end times of the work periods disagree by 0.5s

**Table 9.10** Synthetic reliability data for time motion analysis with mismatching start times

| Observer 1 | | Observer 2 | Total |
|---|---|---|---|
| | Work | Rest | |
| Work | 18 × 5.5s = 99s | 18 × 6s + 18 × 0.5s = 117s | 216s |
| Rest | 18 × 0.5s = 9s | 18 × 18.5s + 18 × 19s = 675s | 684s |
| Total | 108s | 792s | 900s |

are the threshold kappa values between good and acceptable agreement and between acceptable and poor agreement. We should synthesise data that is considered to be at these levels of agreement and from these we can determine the threshold values to use when conducting reliability studies with real data.

First, we will consider the threshold value between acceptable and good strengths of agreement. Consider the first of two observers recording a six-second burst every 45s during a 15-minute observation period. So there are 20 bursts of six seconds and 20 recovery periods of 39s. Now imagine that Observer 2 agrees with 16 of these bursts, failing to record the fifth, tenth, fifteenth and twentieth bursts. This is illustrated in Figure 9.3. Table 9.11 shows the volume of time where the two observers agree

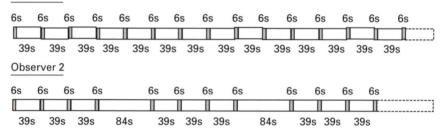

Observer 1

| 6s | 6s | 6s | 6s | 6s | 6s | 6s | 6s | 6s | 6s | 6s | 6s | 6s | 6s | 6s |

| 39s | 39s | 39s | 39s | 39s | 39s | 39s | 39s | 39s | 39s | 39s | 39s | 39s | 39s |

Observer 2

| 6s | 6s | 6s | 6s | | 6s | 6s | 6s | 6s | | 6s | 6s | 6s | 6s |

| 39s | 39s | 39s | 84s | 39s | 39s | 39s | 84s | 39s | 39s | 39s |

**Figure 9.3** Synthetic data for two observers on the threshold of acceptable and good strengths of agreement

**Table 9.11** Synthesising two observers on the threshold of acceptable to good agreement

| *Observer 1* | *Observer 2* | | *Total* |
| | *Work* | *Rest* | |
| --- | --- | --- | --- |
| Work | 16 × 6s = 96s | 4 × 6s = 24s | 120s |
| Rest | 0s | 20 × 39s = 780s | 780s |
| Total | 96s | 804s | 900s |

and disagree about the activity being performed by the player. Both are agreeing that 16 to 20 bursts of six seconds are being performed with one observer recording 39s recoveries while the other records average recoveries of 50.25s. Despite the disagreements, these values are close to the conditions used in Hughes *et al.*'s (2005) laboratory experiment of 6s bursts every 45s and every 55s. The kappa value in this case is 0.8740. If there were mismatches in the agreed bursts reducing the time agreed for these to 5.5s from six seconds, the kappa value would be lower (0.8264). Therefore, based on this example, we might choose a kappa value of 0.8 to be the threshold value between acceptable and good agreement.

To consider the threshold value between acceptable and poor agreement, we will consider 25 bursts performed every 36s during the 15-minute observation period. In reality, the player may be performing six-second bursts with a recovery of 30s in between each. Let us assume that the first observer underestimates the burst duration while the second observer overestimates the burst duration. If the two observers recorded burst durations of four seconds and eight seconds respectively, the level of agreement would not be acceptable simply because one observer is recording twice as much work as the other. If the first observer recorded five-second bursts and the second observer recorded bursts of eight seconds, the disagreement is still serious, but perhaps at the upper end of poor agreement. Burst durations of five seconds and seven seconds would probably be considered close enough to 6s to be an acceptable level of agreement between the observers. So we will use the case where the observers record five-second and eight-second bursts respectively every 36s. This is illustrated in Figure 9.4. Table 9.12 shows the volume of time where they agree and disagree on movement. The kappa value here is 0.7216. If the agreed part of each recorded burst reduced from five seconds to 4.75s due to different burst start times between the two

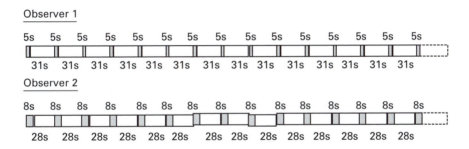

**Figure 9.4** Synthetic data for two observers on the threshold of poor and acceptable strengths of agreement

**Table 9.12** Synthesising two observers on the threshold of poor to acceptable agreement

| Observer 1 | Observer 2 | | Total |
| | Work | Rest | |
| --- | --- | --- | --- |
| Work | 25 × 5s = 125s | 0s | 125s |
| Rest | 25 × 3s = 75s | 25 × 28s = 700s | 775s |
| Total | 200s | 700s | 900s |

observers, then the kappa value would drop to 0.6933. We are now in a much better position to choose threshold values for kappa to be used in reliability studies. Rather than just using the values determined in this exercise, we do need to consider the nature of the sport being observed as some sports are more difficult to observe than others especially if played on a small playing surface requiring many accelerations, decelerations and direction changes. Based on this exercise, we could consider kappa values below 0.7 as being poor, above 0.8 as being good and any in between 0.7 and 0.8 as being acceptable.

This example has used time-motion analysis to convey the concept of meaningful reliability assessment, establishing threshold values for kappa for this particular system that are justified considering energy systems utilised during different types of intermittent high intensity activity. The general approach can be applied in other types of system, such as match analysis systems. Irrespective of whether kappa, percentage or some other reliability statistic is used, we can use synthetic reliability data and deliberately add disagreements of different severities. For example, with the tennis serve system we can create synthetic data where players serve to the left, middle and right of the deuce and advantage courts on first and second serve for realistic percentages of points in those situations. Minor disagreements can be introduced so that the two synthetic observers are at least broadly agreeing on the general service strategy. Major disagreements can then be introduced to represent a situation where the synthetic observers' data portray serving performances of differing strategies. Ultimately, errors need to be synthesised that are on the boundary between good and acceptable agreement and on the boundary between acceptable and poor agreement. The reliability statistics for these synthesised reliability data sets can then be computed and used as threshold values in real reliability studies.

## RELIABILITY OF NUMERICAL DATA

### Numerical data

The events that were discussed previously in the tennis serve and football possession examples are categorical data. The frequencies with which those events occur or the percentage of tennis points or soccer possessions where different combinations of factors apply are numerical, but the raw event data that are gathered are categorical. Similarly, the movement types used in the two-movement and seven-movement time-motion analysis systems are categorical data even though the frequency, mean duration and percentage of match time spent performing these are numbers. In this section of the chapter we discuss the reliability of raw data that are numerical. This will be covered using an example of split times during an 800m race contested by eight athletes. The raw data are the times at which each athlete reached each 100m point during the race. Thus there are 64 timings recorded. The data might have been captured using stopwatches operated by one time-keeper for each athlete during live observation. Alternatively, a race video may be analysed by a single analyst using a stopwatch while watching the race video once for each athlete. A further way the data could be created is by using a computerised system, frequently pausing the video, to identify the times at which each athlete reaches each 100m point during the race.

### Elapsed times and split times

Table 9.13 shows the elapsed times and split times for an 800m race as recorded by two independent observers. There are eight athletes (A to H) whose times have been recorded every 100m during the race. The elapsed time is the time taken from the start of the race for the given athlete to reach the given 100m point. For example, athlete A took 90.01s to reach the 600m point according to Observer 1 and 90.09s according to Observer 2. The split times are times for individual 100m sections of the race. For example, the split times shown at 600m are split times for the 100m section from the 500m point to the 600m point.

### Percentage error

Percentage error can be used with some numerical data using equation (9.1) except V1 and V2 are values of some numerical raw data variables recorded by two observers rather than event frequencies. Some numerical variables are ratio scale variables where values can be 0 or greater. A ratio scale variable is one where 0 represents an absence of the concept being measured. Therefore, distances and times are ratio scale measures because division has meaning; 6s is three times as long as 2s. Percentage error can be used as effectively with such variables as it can with event

Table 9.13 Timing data for an 800m track race

| Distance (m) | Athlete | Elapsed time (s) Observer 1 | Observer 2 | Split time (s) Observer 1 | Observer 2 | Error (s) | Absolute error (s) |
|---|---|---|---|---|---|---|---|
| 100 | A | 14.54 | 14.59 | 14.54 | 14.59 | −0.05 | 0.05 |
| 100 | B | 14.37 | 14.43 | 14.37 | 14.43 | −0.06 | 0.06 |
| 100 | C | 15.54 | 15.62 | 15.54 | 15.62 | −0.08 | 0.08 |
| 100 | D | 15.43 | 15.50 | 15.43 | 15.50 | −0.07 | 0.07 |
| 100 | E | 15.68 | 15.79 | 15.68 | 15.79 | −0.11 | 0.11 |
| 100 | F | 15.23 | 15.37 | 15.23 | 15.37 | −0.14 | 0.14 |
| 100 | G | 14.87 | 15.01 | 14.87 | 15.01 | −0.14 | 0.14 |
| 100 | H | 14.84 | 14.96 | 14.84 | 14.96 | −0.12 | 0.12 |
| 200 | A | 29.88 | 29.94 | 15.34 | 15.35 | −0.01 | 0.01 |
| 200 | B | 29.17 | 29.30 | 14.80 | 14.87 | −0.07 | 0.07 |
| 200 | C | 31.46 | 31.54 | 15.92 | 15.92 | 0.00 | 0.00 |
| 200 | D | 29.85 | 29.94 | 14.42 | 14.44 | −0.02 | 0.02 |
| 200 | E | 31.04 | 31.13 | 15.36 | 15.34 | 0.02 | 0.02 |
| 200 | F | 29.89 | 30.01 | 14.66 | 14.64 | 0.02 | 0.02 |
| 200 | G | 30.40 | 30.49 | 15.53 | 15.48 | 0.05 | 0.05 |
| 200 | H | 28.96 | 29.09 | 14.12 | 14.13 | −0.01 | 0.01 |
| 300 | A | 45.27 | 45.32 | 15.39 | 15.38 | 0.01 | 0.01 |
| 300 | B | 44.56 | 44.65 | 15.39 | 15.35 | 0.04 | 0.04 |
| 300 | C | 47.09 | 47.16 | 15.63 | 15.62 | 0.01 | 0.01 |
| 300 | D | 45.20 | 45.27 | 15.35 | 15.33 | 0.02 | 0.02 |
| 300 | E | 46.24 | 46.33 | 15.20 | 15.20 | 0.00 | 0.00 |
| 300 | F | 44.57 | 44.66 | 14.68 | 14.65 | 0.03 | 0.03 |
| 300 | G | 44.17 | 44.28 | 13.77 | 13.79 | −0.02 | 0.02 |
| 300 | H | 43.10 | 43.19 | 14.14 | 14.10 | 0.04 | 0.04 |
| 400 | A | 59.98 | 60.03 | 14.71 | 14.71 | 0.00 | 0.00 |
| 400 | B | 59.53 | 59.65 | 14.97 | 15.00 | −0.03 | 0.03 |
| 400 | C | 62.32 | 62.39 | 15.23 | 15.23 | 0.00 | 0.00 |
| 400 | D | 59.47 | 59.54 | 14.27 | 14.27 | 0.00 | 0.00 |
| 400 | E | 60.68 | 60.78 | 14.44 | 14.45 | −0.01 | 0.01 |
| 400 | F | 59.93 | 60.02 | 15.36 | 15.36 | 0.00 | 0.00 |
| 400 | G | 58.89 | 58.98 | 14.72 | 14.70 | 0.02 | 0.02 |
| 400 | H | 57.48 | 57.53 | 14.38 | 14.34 | 0.04 | 0.04 |
| 500 | A | 75.22 | 75.29 | 15.24 | 15.26 | −0.02 | 0.02 |
| 500 | B | 73.85 | 73.93 | 14.32 | 14.28 | 0.04 | 0.04 |
| 500 | C | 76.54 | 76.66 | 14.22 | 14.27 | −0.05 | 0.05 |
| 500 | D | 74.60 | 74.73 | 15.13 | 15.19 | −0.06 | 0.06 |
| 500 | E | 75.85 | 75.96 | 15.17 | 15.18 | −0.01 | 0.01 |
| 500 | F | 74.83 | 74.94 | 14.90 | 14.92 | −0.02 | 0.02 |
| 500 | G | 72.67 | 72.76 | 13.78 | 13.78 | 0.00 | 0.00 |
| 500 | H | 71.39 | 71.45 | 13.91 | 13.92 | −0.01 | 0.01 |
| 600 | A | 90.01 | 90.09 | 14.79 | 14.80 | −0.01 | 0.01 |
| 600 | B | 87.50 | 87.56 | 13.65 | 13.63 | 0.02 | 0.02 |
| 600 | C | 90.88 | 90.93 | 14.34 | 14.27 | 0.07 | 0.07 |
| 600 | D | 90.54 | 90.67 | 15.94 | 15.94 | 0.00 | 0.00 |
| 600 | E | 91.43 | 91.53 | 15.58 | 15.57 | 0.01 | 0.01 |
| 600 | F | 89.48 | 89.60 | 14.65 | 14.66 | −0.01 | 0.01 |

# 208

Table 9.13 continued

| Distance (m) | Athlete | Elapsed time (s) | | Split time (s) | | Error (s) | Absolute error (s) |
| | | Observer 1 | Observer 2 | Observer 1 | Observer 2 | | |
| --- | --- | --- | --- | --- | --- | --- | --- |
| 600 | G | 88.16 | 88.22 | 15.49 | 15.46 | 0.03 | 0.03 |
| 600 | H | 86.76 | 86.86 | 15.37 | 15.41 | −0.04 | 0.04 |
| 700 | A | 105.20 | 105.30 | 15.19 | 15.21 | −0.02 | 0.02 |
| 700 | B | 101.33 | 101.40 | 13.83 | 13.84 | −0.01 | 0.01 |
| 700 | C | 106.26 | 106.40 | 15.38 | 15.47 | −0.09 | 0.09 |
| 700 | D | 105.04 | 105.16 | 14.50 | 14.49 | 0.01 | 0.01 |
| 700 | E | 106.84 | 106.93 | 15.41 | 15.40 | 0.01 | 0.01 |
| 700 | F | 104.72 | 104.84 | 15.24 | 15.24 | 0.00 | 0.00 |
| 700 | G | 102.33 | 102.41 | 14.17 | 14.19 | −0.02 | 0.02 |
| 700 | H | 101.31 | 101.41 | 14.55 | 14.55 | 0.00 | 0.00 |
| 800 | A | 120.58 | 120.65 | 15.38 | 15.35 | 0.03 | 0.03 |
| 800 | B | 116.62 | 116.72 | 15.29 | 15.32 | −0.03 | 0.03 |
| 800 | C | 121.54 | 121.68 | 15.28 | 15.28 | 0.00 | 0.00 |
| 800 | D | 120.42 | 120.49 | 15.38 | 15.33 | 0.05 | 0.05 |
| 800 | E | 122.84 | 122.90 | 16.00 | 15.97 | 0.03 | 0.03 |
| 800 | F | 118.96 | 119.06 | 14.24 | 14.22 | 0.02 | 0.02 |
| 800 | G | 116.87 | 116.94 | 14.54 | 14.53 | 0.01 | 0.01 |
| 800 | H | 116.32 | 116.41 | 15.01 | 15.00 | 0.01 | 0.01 |

frequency. However, while split times are ratio scale measures we never see split times of 0s. This means that percentage error values can be misleadingly low because we are dividing by the whole of the mean split time between two observers. Consider the final split time for athlete H where Observers 1 and 2 have recorded 15.01s and 15.00s respectively. The absolute error of 0.01s is equivalent to a percentage error of 0.067 per cent when expressed as a percentage of the mean split time between the two observers of 15.005. Even if a large error in real athletics terms was made, the percentage error would be low. For example, if the observers split times disagreed by 1.00s with an average split of 15.00s, the percentage error would be 6.67 per cent. Many in notational analysis interpret such a percentage error as an acceptable level of inter-observer agreement when testing other systems. However, for split times in sports like track running, percentage error is not recommended. An error of 1.00s is large in real athletic terms.

## Relative reliability

In this example, we determine the reliability for the split times rather than the elapsed times. Simply inspecting the elapsed times that are shown in Table 9.13 reveals that we basically have eight different variables. The 100m times have a different range of values from 200m times, 300m times and so on. A numerical variable has relative reliability if there is a strong positive correlation between the sets of values recorded by two independent observers. If the data in Table 9.14 are stored in Microsoft Excel, then we can simply use the CORREL function to the split times to determine Pearson's coefficient of correlation; in this case r = +0.997. This is a strong positive correlation. We require a higher value for r than we would if correlating two completely different variables. The two observers are recording values for the same variable. Therefore, correlations of +0.9 or greater are needed to conclude acceptable relative reliability. Relative reliability alone is not sufficient to establish the reliability of a method. We could obtain a perfect correlation (r = +1.000) where one observer's set of timings were double the values of the other observer's timings. Therefore, we also need absolute reliability.

## Absolute reliability

Absolute reliability expresses errors in the units of measurement used for the variable of interest (in this case s) or as a ratio. A reliability study of numerical data should always have some measure of absolute reliability. Relative reliability is also important but absolute reliability is essential. The first measure of absolute reliability is mean absolute error which is given by equation (9.3) where V1 and V2 are corresponding values recorded by Observers 1 and 2. N is the number of observations made by each observer. The $\Sigma$ symbol means 'sum' because we need to add up the individual absolute errors when computing the mean absolute error.

$$\text{Mean Abs Error} = (\Sigma_{i=1..N} \mid V1_i - V2_i \mid )/N \tag{9.3}$$

In the example of 800m running, N = 64, and the absolute errors are shown in the far-right column of Table 9.13. The mean absolute error in this case is 0.031s. Those familiar with track athletics may find this an acceptable level of reliability or not. The level of reliability needs to be

210

interpreted in relation to the analytical goals of the study being done. Students should also be creative and informative in describing reliability. For example, mean absolute error could be determined for split times each 100m section of the race as shown in Table 9.14. This shows that the largest errors occur for the first 100m of the race. This could be explained by athletes still running in lanes before they break for the inside lane.

## Systematic bias and random error

A disadvantage of mean absolute error is that it conceals two important components of error within a single value for error. These two components are systematic bias and random error. Systematic bias is a general tendency for one observer to record higher values than the other. This can be represented by the average error which is determined using the errors in the penultimate column of Table 9.13. In this example, the mean error is −0.011s. Therefore, Observer 1 has recorded slightly shorter split times on average than Observer 2. This general tendency for one observer to record higher values than the other is called a systematic bias. It is very slight in this example, but may be more pronounced in analyses of numerical data in other sports.

If we examine the errors in the penultimate column of Table 9.13, we see that they range from −0.14s to +0.07s. Therefore, not all errors are the same as the mean error and there is variability in error values about the systematic bias. This additional error is referred to as random error.

Table 9.14 Mean absolute error values for 100m split times (s) during an 800m race

| Distance (m) | Observer 1 | Observer 2 | Absolute error (s) |
|---|---|---|---|
| 100m | 15.06 | 15.16 | 0.10 |
| 200m | 15.02 | 15.02 | 0.02 |
| 300m | 14.94 | 14.93 | 0.02 |
| 400m | 14.76 | 14.76 | 0.01 |
| 500m | 14.58 | 14.60 | 0.03 |
| 600m | 14.98 | 14.97 | 0.02 |
| 700m | 14.78 | 14.80 | 0.02 |
| 800m | 15.14 | 15.13 | 0.02 |
| Total | 14.91 | 14.92 | 0.03 |

Random error is described using the standard deviation of the error values shown in the penultimate column of Table 9.13. The standard deviation in this case is 0.044s. Two different measures of random error that can be described using this are the standard error of measurement (SEM) and the 95 per cent limits of agreement. The SEM (sometimes referred to as typical error) divides the standard deviation by $\sqrt{2}$ giving 0.031s in this case. The SEM is used with the change in the mean which is the same as the systematic bias. Therefore, we have a change in the mean of $-0.011$s between Observer 1 and Observer 2 and a SEM of 0.031s. If errors are normally distributed then 52 per cent of errors should be within the SEM of the change of the mean. This allows us to consider SEM as an average error.

The 95 per cent limits of agreement cover 95 per cent of errors if they are normally distributed. This requires us to multiply the standard deviation by 1.96 giving 0.087s. The 95 per cent limits of agreement are given by the systematic bias $\pm$ random error. In this case, the 95 per cent limits of agreement are $-0.011 \pm 0.087$s. This means that 95 per cent of errors are between $-0.098$s and $+0.076$s between Observers 1 and 2. These limits should not be considered as an indication of average error. They are the limits outside of which only 5 per cent of errors fall. Whether using change in the mean and SEM or 95 per cent limits of agreement, students should interpret reliability in relation to the analytical goals of system use.

## SUMMARY

Variables used in sports performance analysis need to be valid and reliable. Objectivity can enhance reliability but can also be at the expense of validity. On the other hand, an unreliable variable cannot be valid. Where human operators are part of an analysis system, 100 per cent reliability cannot be guaranteed. Reliability studies are necessary to show the level of reliability of a system. This can be established by analysing the reliability of the input data of a system or by analysing the reliability of its outputs. Inter-operator reliability studies are recommended to show that systems can be used consistently by different personnel. This chapter has covered the use of percentage error as a reliability statistic for event frequencies and numerical measures. Kappa can be used to evaluate the reliability of nominal data when chronologically ordered Event

# 212

Lists exist. Corresponding Event Lists may be of different lengths and so there may be mismatches in the Event Lists that need to be identified during pre-processing of reliability data before kappa is calculated. Kappa can be applied to the frequency or timings of events. There are various reliability statistics that can be used with numerical measures such as split times. Relative reliability can be described using a correlation coefficient while absolute reliability can be described using mean absolute error, change in the mean and SEM or 95 per cent limits of agreement. This chapter has discouraged students from using arbitrary threshold values such as less than 5 per cent error or kappa values greater than 0.6. Instead, we need to consider the threshold values that indicate data are reliable enough in real sports terms. The time-motion analysis system has been used as an example of working out the values of kappa required for acceptable and good reliability. These values are specific to the particular time-motion analysis example. Other applications also need to be considered using synthetic data to establish the level of reliability required before undertaking reliability studies.

# CHAPTER 10

## SCIENTIFIC WRITING IN SPORTS PERFORMANCE ANALYSIS

### INTRODUCTION

This chapter covers different types of report that are produced by sports performance analysis students. The chapter commences with a general section on writing a paper before specifically covering the main reports produced by Level 5 students. Level 5 performance analysis modules typically assess students using two coursework exercises; one on system development focusing on system development and the validity of performance indicators and the other on system testing where the emphasis is on reliability. The chapter briefly covers some other types of report produced by sports performance analysis students. Details of how to undertake a research project leading to a dissertation are covered in the author's 2010 text book (O'Donoghue, 2010). Therefore, this is only covered briefly in the current chapter along with how to prepare an abstract and a poster for conference presentation. There is greater coverage of research proposals as students may have to submit a research proposal during Level 5. The chapter concludes with general guidance on scientific writing and referencing.

### STRUCTURING A SCIENTIFIC PAPER

There are different types of research paper including those describing original research and those reviewing existing research. Original research papers report on research projects where data have been gathered and analysed with conclusions being drawn from the data. Some original research papers report on a series of related studies within a single primary paper. The structure of such papers can vary depending on the number of studies and how they are brought together to provide supporting evidence for any theory being proposed. In the current section of the book we are concerned with papers that describe a single research study that has been completed.

Universities and colleges use different names for the coursework to be submitted by students; essays, reports, papers and so on. Irrespective of the term used, the format of Level 5 coursework follows that of a scientific paper which reports on a research study. Typically, the students are developing a system, applying that system, evaluating it and drawing some conclusions. This is a small-scale version of what happens in the type of sports performance research that is published in academic journals. Therefore, the practical work that has been done by the student is written up in the same way as a scientific paper. The sections required in a paper are:

- Introduction
- Methods
- Results
- Discussion
- Conclusions
- References
- Appendices

Hall (2009) outlined the contents of a scientific paper without including a separate conclusions section. Indeed, many published scientific papers incorporate the conclusions within the discussion section. Students are advised to include a separate conclusions section if there are separate marks allocated for the discussion and conclusions in the particular coursework they are doing. The introduction of a paper should be brief, explaining why the study was done, showing an awareness of previous research and stating what the study adds to our knowledge of the given field (Smith, 2009). The methods section should describe what was done in sufficient detail to allow replication of the study. The methods section of a sports performance analysis paper typically includes an overview of the study's design, definitions of the variables used, a description of the system, reliability of the system, data sources for the study (participants, matches or performances) and data analysis. This order differs from other disciplines of sports science with the data sources covered much later in sports performance analysis. This is because it is necessary to describe the system and establish its reliability before applying it within the main study of the research. The design of the study is an overview of the whole method that concisely tells the reader how the research specifically addresses the purpose and is linked to data analysis. The methods sections within a report being done by Level 5 students might not include all of this information. For example, the reliability results might be included in the results section if the whole purpose of the study was to assess the reliability of one or more systems. In other courseworks done by Level 5 students, reliability assessment might not be required because it is not feasible to train another user to competently use the system in the timescale that has been set.

The results section should show what was found making efficient use of tables, charts and/or other diagrams. The paragraph text within the results section should not merely repeat results shown in tables, charts and diagrams but should describe notable patterns of results. Priebe (2009) suggested that some readers look at the tables, charts and diagrams within results sections before reading the text within the section. Therefore, the tables, charts and other diagrams need to be clear and understandable when considered in isolation from the text. The discussion should explain the results, drawing on relevant literature to support any explanations being made. The main difference between the results section and the discussion section is that the results are describing what was found whereas the discussion is explaining why a study has found what it has found.

## COURSEWORK 1: SYSTEM DEVELOPMENT

### Purpose of the coursework

The first coursework of a Level 5 sports performance analysis module is primarily about validity. The student needs to explore a sport and develop a system allowing some relevant and important aspect of the sport to be recorded and analysed in a way that could provide meaningful information to coaches and players. Ultimately the system needs to be able to provide information that supports decisions of coaches and players. The system is developed and tested by using it to analyse one or more

216

performances. This allows the process and the information produced to be evaluated. The sections of the written report are the same as those in a research paper reporting on original research that have been listed in the previous section of this chapter.

## Introduction

The introduction should commence with a paragraph explaining the overall problem, the sport of interest, the aspect of the sport to be addressed by the system and the purpose of the exercise to develop and evaluate a manual notation system to analyse the given aspect of the given sport.

The remainder of the introduction should discuss the aspect of the sport of interest, justifying its relevance and importance to success in the sport. This typically involves referring to supporting evidence from coaching and professional literature for the sport. Some performance analysis literature can also be referred to where previous research has investigated the chosen aspect of the sport, similar aspects within the sport or the aspect of interest within related sports. However, there may be some students who find that there is little or no sports performance analysis literature covering their sport or the specific aspect of the sport. In situations such as this, the student should follow the review of coaching literature for their sport with a review of sports performance analysis literature, making an argument about how the sports performance analysis techniques they are referring to can be beneficial in the analysis of their chosen sport. For example, a student who is interested in analysing tactical aspects of a new team sport can review how tactics have been analysed in similar team sports. This essentially makes a case that unseen tactical decisions and planning can be inferred from observed behaviour.

## Methods

The purpose of the study that is stated in the introduction tells the reader what was done. The methods section describes how it was done. This should commence with a paragraph that sums up the method without going into detail. This overview should simply state that a system was developed and used to analyse performance in the given sport and provide summary information. The detailed sub-sections of the methods section that follow this are for defining the performance variables used, describing the system and its development and then providing information about the performance(s) that were analysed.

The term 'performance variables' has been used here quite intentionally instead of the term 'performance indicators'. This is because many students will be developing systems that are exploratory, using variables that might not have been used previously and that have not been demonstrated to possess the characteristics of performance indicators. Some students may be able to justify referring to some of their selected variables as performance indicators where there is published research evidence supporting their validity. An area of performance may be valid according to the consensus of practical coaching literature reviewed, but once an operationalised variable is created to represent this aspect of performance, it might not be possible to interpret the variable. Indeed, one of the purposes of the study may be to provide an indication of the range of values that a performance variable has. The preferred order of defining variables is to commence with the system outputs. These act as goal posts for system development and are the variables that could be useful in coach and player decision making. Once these variables are defined, the student should identify the raw data that need to be collected using the system that are necessary to produce the system outputs.

In some cases, it is not necessary to fully define the system output variables as well as the input data. For example, one output variable of a tennis system could be the percentage of points where a player goes to the net. The raw data will include the type of point to be recorded for individual points played. One value of this variable is 'net point'. If net points are included in the definitions of raw input data, then this does not have to be repeated for higher order output variables that are calculated using such raw data. Students are encouraged to use bullet points or tables when defining variables to make them stand out more than they would if included in normal paragraph text.

The information to be produced by the system and the raw data to be entered form the functional requirements for the system. The next sub-section of the methods section should describe the manual notation system that has been developed. This will be a little different from system descriptions that students might have seen in published papers. Often published research in sports performance analysis does not describe the development of a system but simply describes the final system that was used in the research. Indeed, some papers simply define the variables used without showing the system. This allows readers to replicate the study using manual notation systems or systems implemented on commercial video analysis packages. The difference in the report being written by the student is that it is a learning exercise where markers wish to assess the student's ability to conduct pilot studies and choose form layouts to promote efficient data collection and analysis. It is, therefore, recommended that students show any scatter diagrams, event lists or tallying forms used in the system. The system may also include separate forms or graphs for presenting output information. These need to be clear, with visual impact allowing a coach to easily understand the information being conveyed.

The forms alone may not fully inform the reader about the system's operation and, therefore, the procedure with which the forms are used during data collection and subsequent analysis should be described. It is not necessary to show every version of the system as it was revised through repeated pilot work. However, a paragraph on pilot work and the types of changes made to the system and reasons for these changes should be included.

The final sub-section of the methods section describes the performance(s) used to evaluate the system. The decision to use one or more performances depends on the nature of the sport, the duration of performances and the expected number of effort hours that students are expected to devote to the coursework. At the author's university, this coursework is done as part of a 20-credit point module where students are required to do 200 effort hours of Level 5 work including attending lectures, seminars and practical sessions, private study as well as completing the two coursework exercises. If the lectures, seminars, practical sessions and private study require 100 effort hours, then each piece of coursework should require 50 hours to complete. This 50 hours includes the background literature survey, system development, pilot work and write up activity. It is recommended that data collection to test the system should require 5 to 10 hours. This might mean that the student needs to analyse a single soccer match if the system is used while repeatedly pausing the video to record data with follow up analysis activity to produce outputs once the data collection is completed. Alternatively, the system could be used to analyse a series of ten gymnastics performances that are of a shorter duration. It depends on how long it takes to analyse a single performance, but students should ensure that there is a high enough volume of practical data collection and analysis in their coursework in comparison to their classmates.

Having justified the volume of data collection, the student should describe the performances analysed. This includes stating the level, gender and age group of the competition, whether the performances were analysed live or from a video recording. When video recordings are used the student should state whether they personally filmed the performances, used video material provided to students on the module, used public domain broadcast video or accessed video recordings from coaches, athletes or clubs that they are in contact with.

## Results

The results section should provide the results of the analysis as they would be provided to coaches and players. Therefore, the raw data should not be shown, but the summary results should be presented. Any findings supporting the case for the performance variables being potential performance indicators should be highlighted. For example, there may be some performance variables that clearly distinguish between winning and losing performances within an individual or team game. Similarly, there may be some performance variables that clearly distinguish between successful and not so successful gymnastics routines. The results for the given performances should be supported with some commentary about what the system usefully shows.

## Discussion

The important thing to remember in doing coursework like this is that it is sports performance analysis coursework and not coursework about the specific sport of interest. The purpose of the discussion is not to explain the particular performance or why one team was successful and another was not or why a technical performance was flawed or what its strong points were. This is a sports performance analysis coursework and the discussion should be primarily about sports performance analysis issues.

The types of things that can be discussed are the performance variables that were used, usability of the system, sources of inaccuracy and applicability of the system. The performance variables used, their relevance and importance should be discussed. Are they understandable? Is the scale of measurement understood? Are the types of values that we would see for winning and losing teams known? To what extent do the performance variables qualify as performance indicators? This is the student's opportunity to demonstrate their knowledge of performance indicators even if it is only to confirm that their own performance variables fall short of being performance indicators.

In discussing the usability of the system, the student should debate if the system could be used live to record data during a performance. Is there a speed/accuracy trade-off for the system? Might the system need to be used with a subset of the performance variables in order to be used live? This provides the student with the opportunity to demonstrate their knowledge of the distinction between real-time and lapse-time systems, referring to supporting literature when discussing the issues involved. The student should also discuss potential errors that could be made when using the system, identifying sources of inaccuracy when recording performance data. This allows the student to demonstrate knowledge of the types of error that can occur during observational analysis, referring to sports performance analysis literature to support these points.

The type of results that can be produced and the way in which these are presented is a further area of discussion. What is the time scale for producing the results once the performance ends? In the case of a scatter diagram this would be much more immediate than if a sequential system was used. This allows the student to demonstrate knowledge of alternative types of system and their relative advantages and disadvantages. What types of coach decisions can be supported by the information provided? Does the system provide an optimal volume of feedback in a timely manner supporting performance enhancement? Are the types of feedback provided by the system beneficial in helping coaches and players recognise areas requiring attention? These questions should be addressed by using reference to supporting literature from feedback and communication in coaching contexts.

## Conclusions

The conclusions should sum up the main findings of the exercise and the recommendations made. The conclusions section does not continue the discussion.

Any recommendations made about the system and its use should be supported by the findings.

### References and appendices

Referencing will be discussed later in the chapter, but it is important to make sure that readers are aware that a reference list is required at the end of the report. Appendices for this first piece of coursework include data collection forms and any summary analysis forms that have not already been shown in the methods section. One thing that students are advised against is typing up the data entered into manual notation forms. The whole point of using a shorthand notation system is to improve delivery time of system outputs. A practising performance analyst would not waste time typing up tallies that have already been collected and used to produce system outputs.

## COURSEWORK 2: RELIABILITY ASSESSMENT

### Purpose of coursework 1

The first piece of coursework is all about validity and choosing the appropriate aspects of a sport, operationalising them within a system and applying that system. The second piece of coursework is all about reliability. The students use existing system(s) within this exercise, evaluating the consistency with which they can be used by different operators. At Cardiff Metropolitan University, the students do a reliability study of one or more time-motion analysis systems. The reason for choosing this area rather than tactical or technical aspects of sport is that time-motion analysis avoids situations where some students are advantaged by having good understanding of tactical or technical aspects of the sport being used as an example. Time-motion analysis, locomotive movement types, low, moderate and high intensity activity are generic concepts that all students should have a similar understanding of. The students analyse a video of a single player's performance where the video recording follows the player's movement rather than the on-the-ball action. The students typically analyse the performance twice allowing intra-operator agreement of a system to be evaluated. The individual student's data can then be compared with data recorded by a classmate allowing inter-operator agreement to be evaluated. This is done for at least two systems or the same system applied to different sports.

There are variations of the reliability assessment exercise that prevent exactly the same piece of coursework from being repeated in consecutive years. These can be done in a cycle until technology advances allowing a completely different approach to analysing reliability to be used. Some ideas for time-motion analysis reliability studies are:

1. Apply two systems with different interfaces to the analysis of a player's work-rate in a given match using a two-movement classification (work and rest). One system could be implemented in a commercial video editing package where the video is played on the computer used by the student while the other is an implementation (for example in Visual BASIC) without the video on the screen but the system is operated while viewing a video displayed using a data projector.

2. Apply the same system to the analysis of a player's work-rate in a given match using a two-movement classification, but comparing simulated live with lapse-time analysis. This would be done in two different ways. First, users should be allowed to pause, rewind and forward wind the video positioning it to allow the entry of start and end times of work periods. The second way of using the system would involve users playing the video without pausing and entering the start and end of each work period as a simulated real-time observation.

3. A two-movement classification system (work and rest), could be compared with a three-movement (low, moderate and high intensity activity) or seven- movement classification system (stationary, walking, backing, jogging, running, shuffling and game-related activity). Indeed the coursework could compare the three and seven-movement classification systems.

4. The same system could be applied to the analysis of two different sports using two different videos. For example, time-motion analysis may be more challenging in a sport like basketball than in soccer. The comparison of these two different observational tasks using the same system would be an interesting piece of coursework.

In each case, the two alternatives (whether different systems, different sports or different operating conditions) are used twice by the student and twice by a classmate allowing intra- and inter-operator agreement statistics to be determined and compared.

## Introduction

The practical exercise is documented within a written report that follows the structure of a scientific paper. The introduction should provide the reader with a brief background to the exercise, establishing a rationale for the study and stating the purpose of the report. This should not be an exhaustive literature review and students should consider the marking criteria and the percentage of marks awarded for the introduction when deciding how long this should be. This exercise primarily allows assessment of the student's ability to conduct a reliability study. Therefore, the coverage of the time-motion analysis application area should be brief; just enough to state that it is an area of sports performance analysis used to indirectly study the physical demands of sports. The rationale for the study depends on the specific nature of the time-motion tasks being compared. For example, if the same system is to be used in the analysis of two different sports, then the student needs to explain that the intermittent nature of high intensity activity varies between sports making some harder to analyse than others. We cannot assume that because the system is reliable for analysing one sport, that it will be reliable for analysing other sports. Analyses of different sports are different observational tasks with different challenges for observers. If the same video is to be analysed using two different interfaces, whether the differences are in software or hardware, the student needs to provide a rationale based on ergonomics or human-computer interaction. A system could be used reliably when one interface is presented but reliability may be reduced when an alternative interface is used. There is a need to evaluate the level of reliability of the system when each interface is used. The student needs to articulate the need for the study drawing on supporting evidence from published research into reliability evaluation techniques used in sports performance analysis.

Having covered the background and provided a rationale for the study, the student should state the precise purpose of the study. For example, this could be to compare intra- and inter-operator agreement between time-motion analysis systems using a two- movement classification scheme and a seven-movement classification scheme. It is not recommended that the

224

student wastes any words discussing the structure of the report. Readers will already be aware that a report like this will have introductory, methods, results, discussion and conclusions sections.

## Methods

The methods section should describe what was done allowing readers to repeat the study. The methods section includes the design of the study, details of data sources, participants, system development and how reliability statistics were produced. The design of the study shows how the student deliberately set out to address the purpose of the study stated in the introduction. The description of the system used does not provide any information about how often it was used and with what data. Therefore, the student should present an overall research design at the outset of the methods section before going into detail. For example, the student could state that a performance in a given sport was analysed twice by each of two observers using a two- movement classification scheme and twice by each of the two observers using a seven-movement classification scheme. It can then be stated that this allowed comparison of intra-operator agreement and inter-operator agreement for each system.

The data sources are any time-motion video material used in the investigation. The student should describe where these came from, making some comment about duration, the quality of footage and the level of the given sport(s). Some students may include this information under a sub-heading of participants describing the age, level and experience level of the player(s) whose performance(s) were analysed. The sub-section on participants should also describe the experience of the system observers. Readers of the report making decisions about the systems that have been evaluated need some information about the personnel required to achieve the reported reliability. Therefore, the student could state that the observers were undergraduate honours degree students who had been taking a sports performance analysis module over the preceding four months.

In describing the system, the student needs to provide enough information to allow a reader to repeat the study. Where the student has developed the system using a commercially available general purpose video analysis package, the student does not have to repeat information that readers could find elsewhere about the given package. This is a methods section rather than a user manual and students are encouraged to read methods sections of published papers in sports performance analysis and more widely to help understand how to avoid unnecessary detail. A physiology laboratory experiment carrying out a particular test using a stated protocol on named equipment does not need to discuss every click of the mouse or piece of information keyed in on the computer controlling the test. This information can be found in published protocols and user manuals. The researcher does not need to reinvent the wheel in this respect. Instead, they need to describe any warm-up, procedural aspects or other conditions that distinguish their application of the test from the standard test described in existing literature. Similarly in sports performance analysis, we do not need to describe the detailed process of implementing and operating a system in the given video analysis package. The readers may be familiar with these tasks and, if not, they will be capable of accessing this information from elsewhere. The student does need to describe the specific system that they developed using the general purpose video analysis package. What were the events? What types of movement are represented as events? Were system features, such as exclusive linking of events, used in the development of the system?

The data analysis sub-section of the methods describes how the time-motion data collected were processed to produce the required reliability statistics. The student should describe how data in event lists, timelines, and/or summary tables or matrices were processed. There may actually be a feature of the system that calculates the kappa statistic between two sets of data without any further processing required by the student. Some packages still require users to process data themselves in order to produce reliability statistics. Where this is the case, the student needs to describe what system data they used and how it was processed. Data might have been exported into Microsoft Excel where the spreadsheet was programmed to calculate the reliability statistic used. Prior to exporting data, timelines might have been analysed creating intermediate rows showing agreements for given events. All of these steps need to be described. However, the student should avoid showing unnecessary detail of spreadsheet processing. Once again, the student should consider how published research papers describe data processing in sufficient detail to allow readers to repeat the study. For example, the student could state that the total agreed time between observations for each movement type and the total time recorded for each movement type by each observation were used to calculate the proportion of time where a pair of observations agreed ($P_0$) and the proportion of time where they would be expected to agree by chance ($P_C$), allowing kappa to be calculated. This is sufficient detail to allow readers to program spreadsheets themselves using published equations for kappa, $P_0$ and $P_C$.

## Results

The results should report what was found delaying any explanation of the findings until the discussion section. The results should be concise, making effective use of tables and charts. Table 10.1 is an example of how the results of a reliability study can be presented. The student will have already named the observations A1, A2, B1 and B2 (for example). A1 and A2 can be used to name the student's first and second analyses of the time-motion video respectively while B1 and B2 can be used to represent the other observer's first and second analyses. The text of the results section should refer to any tables or charts that are included, describing broadly what was found. The student should avoid repeating the exact same values in text that we can already see in the table. The text of the results needs to be more abstract in describing what was found. For example, the student could state that there was greater intra-operator agreement than inter-operator agreement for both systems. Similarly, inter-operator agreement improved from the first analysis of the time-motion video to the second analysis for both systems.

Students should not show unnecessary intermediate data, screen dumps of spreadsheets or system outputs showing individual reliability results for single pairs of analyses. This is not done in published research papers.

Table 10.1 Strength of intra- and inter-operator agreement for the two systems (values in parentheses are the strengths of agreement represented by the kappa values according to Altman (1991: 404))

| Comparison | 2-movement classification | 7-movement classification |
|---|---|---|
| *Intra-operator greement* | | |
| A1 v A2 | 0.82 (very good) | 0.57 (moderate) |
| | | |
| *Inter-operator agreement* | | |
| A1 v B1 | 0.64 (good) | 0.35 (fair) |
| A1 v B2 | 0.66 (good) | 0.46 (moderate) |
| A2 v B1 | 0.62 (good) | 0.31 (fair) |
| A2 v B2 | 0.78 (good) | 0.53 (moderate) |

Students should also avoid showing the exact same results in both tables and charts. This can actually confuse the reader who will be trying to work out what is different between the findings shown in the table and the chart.

The reliability statistics can be interpreted in the results section. For example, Table 10.1 shows that the kappa values for the two-movement classification system represent good to very good strengths of agreement while the kappa values achieved using the seven-movement classification system are interpreted as fair to moderate. Including these interpretations in parentheses in the table is an efficient use of space and avoids cumbersome sentences interpreting the kappa values. There is no need for students to include Altman's full classification table once Altman's classification has been referred to. Indeed readers of the student's report who are familiar with sports performance analysis will already be familiar with the use and interpretation of kappa within reliability studies.

## Discussion

The discussion should explain the findings rather than merely repeating them. In considering the results in Table 10.1, the student needs to ask why they achieved the range of kappa values they did when performing the time-motion analysis tasks. Why was there a greater strength of intra-operator agreement than inter-operator agreement for both systems? Why was there an improvement in inter-operator agreement from the first analysis to the second analysis of the time-motion video. Why was the reliability of the two-movement classification system higher than that of the seven- movement classification system? The student should think about each of these questions, what the explanations may be and what evidence they can draw on from published research to support these explanations. Once this has been done, the student is in a much better position to plan the discussion section and identify the paragraphs to be included.

The explanations of the reliability levels found may be due to the inter-mittent nature of the movement performed in the given sport, the limited experience of the observers as well as definitional, perceptual and data entry errors (James *et al.*, 2002). The student could refer to published time-motion studies comparing kappa values to those achieved in their

228

own exercise. The differences in kappa values between the studies may be explained by the greater density of work of shorter work periods in the sport analysed in one of the studies. The guidelines for what activity should be recorded as work and rest within a two-movement classification will have been vague compared to many other variables used in sports performance analysis. It is not really possible to operationalise these terms to the extent that independent observers will have an identical understanding of what to record as work and rest in all possible situations. There are many grey areas during observation of player movement where an observer will be uncertain of whether to classify it as work or rest and yet needs to make a decision and enter data. This is an example of a definitional error where the same guidelines, presented in words, are interpreted differently by independent observers when observing time-motion video footage.

Perceptual errors are where system operators have an understanding of the data entry task and what they are classifying as work and rest in general, but misclassify behaviour in specific situations. There may be behaviour that required high intensity effort for the player under observation that was not recognised by an observer. Similarly, there may be times when the observer perceives movement to require high intensity effort but the player might actually have performed the behaviour at a lower intensity. The student should give examples of particular behaviours observed in the sport that could be misclassified. General points about the limitations of observational analysis for indirectly analysing the intensity of activity can also be made when discussing perceptual errors and students should support this with reference to alternative more direct measures that could be made.

Data entry errors are where observers correctly classify behaviour but press an incorrect key when entering data. The students should seek to explain this in terms of the usability of the system interface as well as other explanations such as observer fatigue. A more common example of data entry error is delayed data entry due to the observer being taken by surprise by the player under observation changing movement type. It is common in many sports for players to use deception and surprise to gain an advantage over opponents. If they can achieve this against expert opponents in the given sport, they will also be able to take observers who are not as familiar with the sport by surprise. This could be through sudden accelerations or decelerations. The student should refer to relevant coaching literature in the given sport(s) to support this point.

In considering the overall level of reliability, the student should assess whether the system is fit for purpose. This involves looking at system outputs rather than relying solely on the reliability statistics. For example, we might have a situation where a kappa value is fair or moderate and yet the outputs produced by the pair of analyses broadly agree that the sport involves intermittent high intensity activity performed on a backdrop of low intensity movement. Alternatively, we may have good strengths of agreement between observations where inspection of the system outputs shows serious disagreements between the observations in real sports terms. The outputs of interest are the number of work periods, the mean duration of those work periods, the mean duration of recovery periods and the percentage of observation time spent performing work. These could indicate differing mixes of energy systems being used despite the fact that the two observations were of the same performance and the reliability statistic is interpreted as a good strength of agreement. This allows the student to discuss the suitability of the reliability statistic itself for this type of application. Is kappa suitable for evaluating reliability of time-motion analysis systems? Is percentage error or other alternative reliability statistics valid for such an application? Is the interpretation of kappa proposed by Altman (1991: 404) for applied medical science research suitable in sports performance analysis? In discussing the work to rest ratios produced by different observations, the students should avoid going into too much detail about physiology and be mindful that this is a coursework for a sports performance analysis module rather than a physiology module.

Differences between observers may be reflected in higher intra-operator agreement than inter-operator agreement. Students should find it relatively easy to explain that while individuals may be able to apply the tasks consistently, their perceptions of effort may differ to other people. This may be due to the observers coming from different sporting backgrounds.

Changes in inter-operator agreement from the first to second analyses of the time-motion video should be explained in terms of user training effects or increased familiarity with the particular performance. When comparing the two different tasks, students should not only explain why they have similar or differing levels of reliability, but also raise implications for time-motion analysis research. For example, there may be a trade-off between having data on individual types of low and high intensity activity in a seven-movement classification with a greater level of reliability when using a two-movement classification.

# 230

## Conclusions

The conclusions should sum up what was found and make recommendations that are supported by the findings. The conclusions should be brief, covering the main findings. Any recommendations should be based on what was found not on what the student might have preferred to find. For example, if a student finds a greater level of inter-operator agreement and intra-operator agreement when using the seven-movement classification than the two-movement classification, they should not discuss this by saying

> the study found that the seven-movement classification system was more reliable but it is recommended that time-motion studies use the two-movement classification system instead because the combining of different types of work and different types of rest reduces the scope for error.

The student should not worry if it is necessary to conclude that the system should not be used in time-motion investigations with operators of the level of training that were used in the current study. If the results have shown that reliability is not acceptable, then this is the conclusion and it is a valid finding about the system when used for the task of analysing the given sport(s).

## OTHER TYPES OF REPORT

### Dissertation proposal

This section of the chapter covers some other types of report that students produce. These are the dissertation and other reports related to the dissertation. The dissertation proposal is important to Level 5 students because they may be required to submit a dissertation proposal during Level 5. The dissertation, itself, is done in Level 6 and is an independent research project requiring sustained independent effort. For example, at the author's university, it is worth 40 UK credit points and, therefore, requires 400 effort hours of Level 6 work. It is essential that the student puts considerable thought into the research area that they will choose to engage with for their dissertation. The area will need to be of interest to the student, of general interest, an area of strength for the student as well as feasible. Other factors influencing the choice of research topic are time constraints, resources and programme regulations (Walliman, 2004: 24–35). Walliman (2004: 70–75) outlined the contents of a research proposal which include the background, defining the research problem, the main concepts and variables, methods, expected outcomes and a programme of research.

The background section introduces the topic of interest before critically reviewing relevant literature. The review of literature should demonstrate that the student has undertaken background reading, covering the most important research. The student should demonstrate knowledge of relevant theoretical concepts, academic debate within the topic as well as gaps that exist in our knowledge of the given topic. This provides a rationale for the proposed study which should be supported by the justification of the importance of the proposed research.

The statement of the research problem should specify what the student will study in terms of the sport of interest, aspect of the sport, variables to be used and the scope of the study. The scope of the study restricts the age group and level of the sport within the study. For example, a study of soccer tactics might be restricted to the FIFA (Fédération Internationale de Football Association) 2014 World Cup. The variables include any independent and dependent variables of interest. For example, we may hypothesise that the frequency and percentage conversion rates for certain skills differ between playing positions in soccer. In this case, playing position is the independent variable and the frequency and conversion rate variables are the dependent variables. In a quantitative sports performance analysis investigation, we can decide on the format of results before collecting any data or even devising methods. These expected outcomes are related to the purpose of the study. We will not know what values will be displayed on charts or within tables, but if we understand our research question, we can at least know what charts and tables we will produce.

Having established what will be studied, the proposal needs to describe how the research will be done. This is covered in the methods section. There are two main differences between the methods section of a research proposal and the methods section of a paper describing completed research. First, the research proposal is written in the future tense. Second, the full detail of the performance analysis system to be used in the research is not necessarily provided. Part of the Level 6 research project will be to develop the system and test its reliability before applying it to the main research study. Students should be able to state what statistical tests they are going to use during data analysis. Typically sports performance analysis dissertations use non-parametric procedures. So if we understand the purpose of our study, the independent and dependent variables, then we can state the statistical tests that will be used to answer the research question. For example, if we are comparing performance in two different levels of a sport in terms of some numerical dependent variables we know we should use a Mann-Whitney U test.

The appendices of a dissertation proposal should include a programme of research and ethics documentation. The programme of research shows the various activities involved in the research project including system development, data collection, background reading and chapter writing. Anything that takes time should be included. There may be a critical path of activity that can be identified on which the timely completion of the project depends. Some activities can run in parallel with others whereas others may be in sequence. For example, we cannot discuss the results until we have analysed the data and we cannot analyse the data until they have been collected.

Many sports performance analysis dissertations do not have ethical concerns and use public domain data allowing approval by protocol. This means that there may be a class of project that is restricted to the analysis of public domain video that has been approved. This allows any research project to be approved if it can be demonstrated to operate according to this protocol. Projects involving the students doing their own filming or other areas of ethical concern need to be accompanied by ethics applications written well enough to permit an ethics committee to make a decision on the research.

## The dissertation

The dissertation itself is a report on the Level 6 research project once it is completed. This is much larger than a research paper and includes separate introduction and literature review chapters. The review of literature is a more exhaustive coverage of relevant literature than one might expect in a published research paper. It typically moves from the broad topic area funnelling into the specific published research most related to the student's study. Most sports performance analysis studies are empirical studies and so the remaining chapters of the thesis correspond to sections of a research paper. The conclusions are typically longer in a dissertation and the chapter includes main conclusions, practical recommendations and direction for future research. The research project does involve a considerable volume of work, but it is also very satisfying for a student to have undertaken a research project themselves and produced previously unknown knowledge about sports performance.

## A conference abstract

Student research projects sometimes lead to publication in a journal or presentation at a conference. The first thing to say about this is that the student should focus on their programme of study and go for every mark in every module. The distraction of getting the dissertation research accepted for conference presentation or by a journal is time consuming at a critical stage of the student's programme of study. Some outstanding students do make the extra commitment to getting their research published without it affecting their degree outcome. However, the administrative overheads of submitting an abstract or paper are often best left to the supervisor. Once the dissertation has been submitted, the supervisor can produce a one page abstract from the material in the dissertation or cut the dissertation down to the size of a journal paper. This is best done after the dissertation has been submitted rather than the student benefiting from undue staff input to the student's independent research prior to submission. The student is usually named as first author as the person who did the research, with the supervisor's contribution warranting their inclusion as a second author. The abstract is a synopsis of the whole study stating what the purpose was, what was done and what was found. It contains very brief information on the background, methods, results and conclusions (Gustavii, 2008: 59). However, authors should always follow the specific instructions for abstracts being submitted to the particular conference. The methods paragraph needs to broadly state what was done without going into full details of a methods section. This might simply state that a computerised match analysis system was used and stating the number of matches used from different tournaments. Abstracts in sports performance analysis often make effective use of a summary table of the main results at the bottom. Examples of sports performance analysis abstracts can be found in an Annex of the

234

*International Journal of Performance Analysis of Sport* (Volume 12 Number 3 pages 643–839). These are abstracts from the World Congress of Performance Analysis of Sport held at Worcester in July 2012.

## A conference poster

An abstract for a conference may be accepted for podium presentation or poster presentation. Both are considered of equal value but the podium presentation has the advantages that the author(s) can prepare their slides right up until the day before presentation and only need to bring the presentation on a USB drive to the conference. The poster needs to be printed in advance of travelling to the conference and needs to be carried along with the authors' other luggage to and from the conference. The printing of a poster can be expensive, especially if several posters are being presented by a research team. Therefore, the authors should thoroughly check the electronic version of the poster before getting it printed. The poster is not a paper but a synopsis (Matthews and Matthews, 2008: 99). A good poster can contain a little more text than the abstract, but can be accompanied by key tables, charts and other diagrams that have visual impact. At the World Congress of Performance Analysis of Sport, authors are given two to three minutes to present their research with time for two or three questions. This means that the authors do not need to include every word of their presentation on the poster itself. The poster should also be able to stand alone as other delegates may read it during breaks between conference sessions.

## GENERAL GUIDANCE ON SCIENTIFIC WRITING

### Use of language, grammar, spelling and punctuation

In writing a scientific report, the student should consider why they are writing and who the audience is (Creme and Lea, 2008: 5). The student has been given a practical task to do which might have been done very well but it also needs to be reported well. The student needs to convey the message about what they have done, what they have found and their understanding of the academic context of the exercise. The report is about a study that has been completed and, therefore, the methods and results should be described in the past tense. When referring to previous investigations, authors should also use the past tense to describe what was done and what was found. In scientific reports, the student should avoid using the words 'I' and 'we'. Rather than stating 'I watched a 90 minute football match', the student should state 'A 90 minute football match was observed'. In reflective reports on work experience, for example, the words 'I' and 'we' can be used.

When referring to previous research, students should concentrate on what was found and be critical of the methods used where there are limitations. The real evidence of a research study is in the findings rather than speculative comments made in introduction or discussion sections. Students should avoid statements like 'the researchers believe', 'the researcher's think' and 'the researchers suggested'. In quantitative research, the conclusions are supported by the data. Therefore, it is better to say 'the study found', 'the study revealed' or 'the study showed'. The review of literature should be balanced recognising the strengths and limitations of previous research studies.

Students should use gender neutral language avoiding sexist terms (Walliman, 2004: 151). In sports performance analysis, we should refer to camera operators rather than cameramen. Correct grammar, spelling and punctuation should be used within reports to avoid losing marks for presentation. The structure of the paper should be clear using subheadings to make the structure obvious. Information should be presented in a convenient order and in manageable paragraphs with clear, simple sentences (Cooter, 2009).

**Numerical results**

In presenting numerical results, sports performance analysts often need to present frequencies as well as percentages, particularly where the percentages may come from small numbers. For example, 75 per cent is certainly greater than 60 per cent but if the 75 per cent refers to 3 out of 4 tackles that are made successfully in one area of the pitch compared with 12 out of 20 in another area of the pitch, then it is better to include the frequencies in the results as well (3/4 = 75 per cent and 12/20 = 60 per cent). A common mistake made by sports performance analysis students is failing to use SI units. They should use 's' instead of 'seconds' and 'm' instead of 'metres'.

When presenting levels of significance, students should not state 'p < 0.000'. p is a probability and cannot be less than 0. A statistics package may report significance to three decimal places as 0.000. In such cases, 'p = 0.000' is correct to three decimal places, but the author usually reports such values as p < 0.001 just to re-enforce the point that the p value is not actually zero.

## Charts

Figure 10.1 is an example of a line graph used to compare the strategies of 800m athletes who were attempting an 800m/1,500m 'double' with those who were only attempting the 800m. This can be used to compare pacing strategies of the two types of athlete in early rounds and the final. Line graphs are suitable where the variable on the horizontal axis and the dependent variable (on the vertical axis) are both measured on continuous scales. Note that the variable on the horizontal axis in this particular chart is not the independent variable within the study. The independent

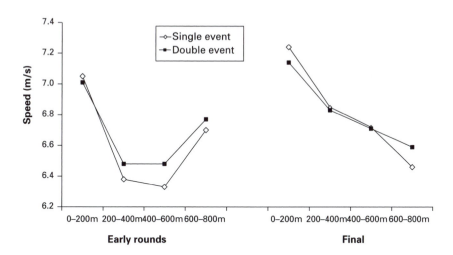

**Figure 10.1** Running speed of the finalists of the women's 800m Olympic Games 2004 during the early rounds and later rounds comparing those athletes who attempted the 800m / 1,500m double (n=3) with the athletes who only did the 800m (n=5). Data from Brown (2005)

variable is the type of athlete (an athlete attempting the 800m/1,500m double or an athlete doing a single event). The horizontal axis summarises distance within the race as being in particular 200m sections. This can still be shown in a line graph because one 200m section of a race is immediately followed by another. In producing line graphs, the student should make them as clear as possible and not clutter the chart with too many different lines. In this case, the early rounds have been combined to simplify the chart and the early round data have been shown in a different area of the chart from the final. This avoids the four lines overlapping each other if the data from the two types of race had been kept together. Error bars could have been used to show variability about the mean speeds. The vertical axis used for speed has used an appropriate range of values that has not exaggerated any differences. The speeds of 6.2 and 7.4m.s$^{-1}$ correspond to 400m lap times of 54.1s and 64.5s respectively. This would be a familiar range of paces one would expect to see for 800m running at the given standard. If the vertical axis used all values from 0m.s$^{-1}$ to 7.4m.s$^{-1}$ it would be misleading by making the races look even paced due to a large empty area of the graph that represents speeds of less than 5m.s$^{-1}$ that have been seen in the women's marathon. Figure headings should appear below charts and any other diagrams used.

Column charts are used when the variable on the horizontal axis is a categorical variable, such as a grouping variable or condition under which performances are observed. Figure 10.2 shows an example of a column chart that compares rally durations in Grand Slam singles tennis between two different eras. The period 1997–9 was prior to surface grading and the introduction of the Type 1 and Type 3 balls while 2007 was after this change. The use of '&' and '$' symbols within the column chart shows significant differences between pairs of tournaments within eras and genders. Augmenting these results to the descriptive results displayed in the chart saves a lot of paragraph text. A line graph here would not be appropriate because there are four different tournaments rather than tournaments being on a continuous numerical scale. There is a case that could be made for using coefficient of friction or coefficient of restitution of court surfaces as numerical variables within studies. However, this is not what has been done here and so a column chart should be used rather than a line graph. The columns represent mean values while the error columns represent standard deviations. There are two means involved here. The dependent variable is mean rally duration within a match but the bars of Figure 10.2 represent the mean of these means

238

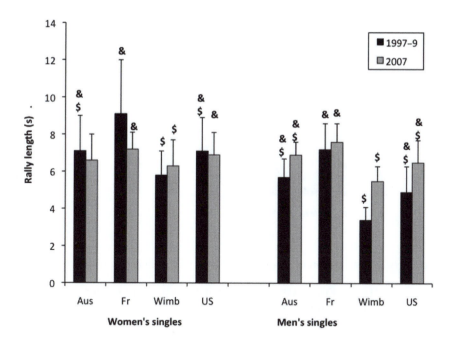

**Figure 10.2** Mean rally duration at Grand Slam tennis tournaments in 1997–9 and 2007 (Aus: Australian Open, Fr: French Open, Wimb: Wimbledon, US: US Open, &: Mann-Whitney U tests revealed significant difference from Wimbledon (p < 0.017); $ Mann-Whitney U tests revealed significant difference from French Open (p < 0.017)). Data from Over and O'Donoghue (2008)

within particular samples of matches. This is a clustered column chart because there are two types of column, one for each era. A common mistake made by students when doing column charts is including a legend where all of the columns are the same colour. For example, if the example in Figure 10.2 just showed the four columns for women's singles in 2007, we would not need a legend because the tournament name is indicated on the horizontal axis.

Figure 10.3 is an example of a compound column chart that shows the distribution of point types at the four Grand Slam tennis tournaments. A compound column chart stacks columns on top of each other allowing readers to see the total of the values as well as individual values. In Figure 10.3, the percentage of points that are of each type are added

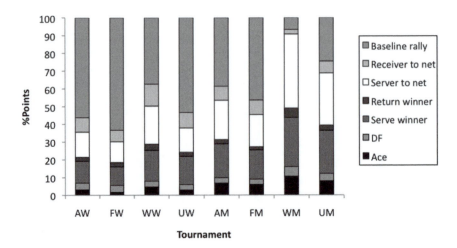

**Figure 10.3** Distribution of points at the four Grand Slam tennis tournaments (A: Australian Open, F: French Open, W: Wimbledon, U: US Open, W: Women's Singles, M: Men's Singles). Data from O'Donoghue and Ingram (2001)

together giving a total of 100 per cent. There are other occasions where the totals shown in a compound column chart come to different values. This is a more concise presentation than using eight separate pie charts. Where the totals are different, separate pie charts would actually conceal these differences from the readers. There is a role for pie charts in presenting sports performance results, especially where a single pie chart shows the distribution of some nominal variable. However, multiple pie charts should not be used where a single table or chart could present the results more concisely.

**Tables**

Tables have advantages and disadvantages over charts. The main advantage of using tables is that we can see actual values for descriptive statistics, whether they are means with accompanying standard deviations or medians and inter-quartile ranges. It is possible for values to be superimposed on charts, but where there are a lot of small columns in a column chart (for example in Figure 10.3), the values would be difficult to include. A further advantage is that tables are good at presenting vari-

240

ables that are measured using different ranges of values. If a variable such as distance covered by soccer players (in the order of 10,000m) and percentage of match time spent moving at $7m.s^{-1}$ or faster (usually less than 3 per cent) were shown in the same column chart, the columns for the percentage of match time spent moving at $7m.s^{-1}$ would be very small.

A disadvantage of tables is that they do not have the visual impact of well-presented charts. Table 10.2 is an example of a table which shows the effect of opposition quality on three performance variables in tennis. The percentage of points won on first and second serve are outcome indicators while the percentage of points where players went to the net is an indicator of tactics. Player quality is examined by considering three types of players based on their world rankings. This table not only shows descriptive statistics (mean±SD) for the nine different types of performance, but also shows inferential statistics using a column for the main test of opposition effect (Kruskal-Wallis H test) and symbols to highlight differences between pairs of performances (Mann-Whitney U test). Unlike figure headings, table headings appear above tables.

Table 10.2 Performances of female tennis players in matches at Grand Slam singles tournaments (mean±SD)

| Player world ranking Performance Indicator | Opponent world ranking | | | Kruskal Wallis H test |
|---|---|---|---|---|
| | 1 to 20 (n=42) | 21 to 75 (n=57) | 76 or lower (n=52) | |
| *Ranked 1 to 20* | | | | |
| % Won on 1st serve | 59.8±10.8 &^ | 71.8±9.7 | 72.0±10.3 | p < 0.001 |
| % Won on 2nd serve | 47.8±11.7 | 50.3±11.5 | 51.8±11.1 | p = 0.130 |
| % Net points played | 11.5±6.2 | 12.3±6.4 | 12.4±6.8 | p = 0.393 |
| *Ranked 21 to 75* | | | | |
| % Won on 1st serve | 54.9±11.2 &^ | 61.9±12.2 | 64.0±9.0 | p < 0.001 |
| % Won on 2nd serve | 41.7±11.9 ^ | 44.5±12.4 | 49.9±12.9 | p = 0.019 |
| % Net points played | 9.2±5.7 | 7.4±6.2 | 7.0±5.7 | p = 0.090 |
| *Ranked 76 or lower* | | | | |
| % Won on 1st serve | 57.0±10.0 ^ | 57.1±12.2 ^ | 63.6±9.3 | p = 0.004 |
| % Won on 2nd serve | 37.1±9.8 ^ | 41.5±11.6 | 46.4±11.7 | p < 0.001 |
| % Net points played | 9.4±5.3 ^ | 7.9±7.6 ^ | 5.0±6.5 | p < 0.001 |

Notes: & Mann-Whitney U test revealed significant difference to match against opponent ranked 21 to 75 (p < 0.017).
^ Mann-Whitney U test revealed significant difference to match against opponent ranked outside World's top 75 (p < 0.017).

Students should use a consistent number of decimal places within rows (or columns) used for a given variable. For example, in Table 10.2, numbers like 72.0, 64.0, 9.0, and 7.0 are presented instead of 72, 64, 9 and 7.

A table has a title, headings and body as shown in Table 10.2. When developing a table such as Table 10.2, the student has a choice as to whether to place the variables in columns of rows. The current example has used rows. The opponent groupings have been shown as columns with row clusters used for each player grouping. Where a table is used to present the descriptive results for variables within different samples (groups or conditions), the student could use rows for the variables and columns for the samples or vice versa. The author has arranged tables both ways and the decision is usually based on being able to fit the number of columns into the width of the page. There are other tables that have values of variables in both rows and columns. For example Tables 9.3(a), 9.3(b), 9.5, 9.6, 9.7, 9.8 and 9.9, in Chapter 9, cross-tabulate values of a nominal variable with themselves to show the level of agreement between observations. There are examples of very large tables used to summarise literature within review articles (MacKenzie and Cushion, 2012) and research studies the results of which are included in meta-analyses (Cobley *et al.*, 2009). These are justified as they provide useful summaries of the literature in terms of sample sizes, variables used and significance or effect sizes of findings. There are other times where tables may be grossly oversized and this should be avoided (Matthews and Matthews, 2008: 61).

### Referencing

Students should use references to supporting literature in both the introduction to a report as well as the discussion section. The student should use the referencing system recommended by their university or college and this should be used consistently and correctly. Students should include references to original research articles published in peer reviewed research journals. Additional references to text books are also important especially where these are used to justify areas of performance being analysed. Book chapters can also be referred to especially if the book is a published conference proceedings where the chapters are reporting on completed studies that were presented at the conference.

242

The Science and Racket Sports and Science and Football series published by Routledge are examples of such conference proceedings. All references used in the report should be included in the reference list at the end of the report. Similarly each reference in the reference list should be used at least once in the text of the report. The reference list should be in alphabetical order of author surname. Where more than one item of work by the same author has been referred to, the author's single author work should be listed first in date order followed by papers co-authored by the author as first named author. The author's papers with a single co-author precede those with more than one co-author.

## Planning, writing, reviewing and rewriting

Word processing has changed the way we write (Creme and Lea, 2008: 10) allowing efficient editing of reports. This allows skeletal plans for reports to be produced with section text added once the student understands how the overall report will fit together. Ideas for content that come to mind during brainstorming can be entered into a document under construction (Creme and Lea, 2008: 19–21). These segments of text can then be placed in an order and linked together in a way that outlines an argument. As the report evolves, the student should read sections and make any amendments needed to communicate the message to the reader more effectively. The use of cut and paste does help the gradual development of a report. However, students should not paste material into their report from copyrighted published sources. Where students paste material from published sources into their report, it is plagiarism. The student might have intended to reword the pasted text and acknowledge the source, but if the student forgets what they wrote and what was pasted in from published material, they commit plagiarism. This will be detected by systems such as Turnitin and the student will be penalised.

## SUMMARY

Communication is essential in all areas of science including sports performance analysis and coaching science. If an academic makes a scientific discovery about sports performance, it will be lost unless it can be communicated effectively in a research report. Similarly, if a practising performance analyst identifies an area of performance requiring attention from athletes or teams they are working with, this will only lead to performance enhancement if the information is presented effectively allowing decisions about preparation and competition to be made by coaches and athletes. Marking schemes often give marks for different report sections without any additional marks for practical exercises that are being written about. However, students should not undervalue the practical task to be done. The report cannot be written about the practical exercise unless the practical exercise has been done. This is no different from what happens when students write laboratory reports for physiology and biomechanics experiments.

The current chapter has intentionally focused on the reporting of the main pieces of coursework to be undertaken by Level 5 sports performance analysis students. These follow the typical structure of a scientific research paper with introduction, methods, results, discussion and conclusion sections. General guidance on a number of areas of scientific writing has also been given. These include the use of language, grammar, presenting charts, presenting tables and referencing. There is also a section on scientific writing in general covering the use of language, tables, diagrams and referencing.

# REFERENCES

Altman, D.G. (1991) *Practical Statistics for Medical Research*, London: Chapman & Hall.

Attrill, M.J., Gresty, K.A., Hill, R., Barton, R.A. (2008) 'Red shirt colour is associated with long-term team success in English football', *Journal of Sports Sciences*, 26: 577–82.

Bangsbo, J., Nørregaard, L. and Thorsøe, F. (1991) 'Activity profile of professional soccer', *Canadian Journal of Sports Sciences*, 16: 110–6.

Bartlett, R.M. (1999) *Sports Biomechanics: reducing injury and improving performance*, London: Routledge.

Bartlett, R.M. (2002) 'Performance analysis: can bringing together biomechanics and notational analysis benefit coaches?', *International Journal of Performance Analysis in Sport*, 1: 122–6.

Bloomfield, J., Polman, R. and O'Donoghue, P.G. (2004) 'The Bloomfield Movement Classification: movement analysis of individual players in dynamic movement sports', *International Journal of Performance Analysis of Sport*, 4(2): 20–31.

Bloomfield, J., Polman, R. and O'Donoghue, P.G. (2007), 'Physical demands of different positions in FA Premier League Soccer', *Journal of Sports Science and Medicine*, 6: 63–70.

Bracewell, P.J., Meyer, D. and Ganesh, S. (2003) 'Creating and monitoring meaningful individual rugby ratings', *Research Letters in the Information and Mathematical Sciences*, 4: 19–22.

Brown, E. (2005) 'Running strategy of female middle distance runners attempting the 800m and 1500m "Double" at a major championship: a performance analysis and qualitative investigation', *International Journal of Performance Analysis of Sport*, 5(3): 73–88.

Brown, E. and O'Donoghue, P.G. (2006) Analysis of performance in running events (pp. 361–72), Cardiff: CPA Press, UWIC.

Brown, E. and O'Donoghue, P.G. (2008) 'A split screen system to analyse coach behaviour: a case report of coaching practice', *International Journal of Computer Science in Sport*, 7(1): 4–17.

Bruggerman, G-P. and Glad, B. (1990) 'Time analysis of sprint events'. In G-P. Bruggerman and B. Glad (eds), *Scientific Research into the Games of the XXIVth Olympiad Seoul 1988, Final Report* (pp. 91–131), Monaco: IAF/IAAF.

Bruggeman, G-P., Koszewski, D. and Muller, H. (1999) *Biomechanical Research Project: Athens 1997 – Final Report*, International Athletic Federation, Oxford, UK: Meyer and Meyer Sport.

Campos, J. (2013) 'Field athletics'. In T. McGarry, P.G. O'Donoghue and J. Sampaio (eds), *Routledge Handbook of Sports Performance Analysis* (pp. 464–74), London: Routledge.

Carling, C. and Bloomfield, J. (2013) 'Time-motion analysis'. In T. McGarry, P.G. O'Donoghue and J. Sampaio (eds), *Routledge Handbook of Sports Performance Analysis* (pp. 283–96), London: Routledge.

Carling, C., Bloomfield, J., Nelson, L. and Reilly, T. (2008) 'The role of motion analysis in elite soccer: contemporary performance measurement techniques and work rate data', *Sports Medicine*, 38: 839–62.

Choi, H., O'Donoghue, P.G. and Hughes, M. (2006a) 'A study of team performance indicators by separated time scale using a real-time analysis technique within English national basketball league'. In H. Dancs, M. Hughes and P.G. O'Donoghue (eds), *Performance Analysis of Sport 7* (pp. 138–41), Cardiff: CPA Press, UWIC.

Choi, H., Reed, D., O'Donoghue, P.G. and Hughes, M. (2006b) 'The valid numbers of performance indicators for real-time analysis using prediction models within men's singles in 2005 Wimbledon Tennis Championship'. In H. Dancs, M. Hughes and P.G. O'Donoghue (eds), *Performance Analysis of Sport 7* (pp. 220–6), Cardiff: CPA Press, UWIC.

Claudio, R. and Dimas, P. (1995) 'Pen based computing: breakthrough in match observation and analysis', ThirdWorld Congress of Science and Football, Cardiff, UK, 9–13 April.

Coalter, A., Ingram, B., McCrorry, P., O'Donoghue, P.G. and Scott, M. (1998) 'A comparison of alternative operation schemes for the computerised scoring system for amateur boxing', *Journal of Sports Sciences*, 16: 16–7.

Cobley, S., Baker, J., Wattie, N. and McKenna, J. (2009) 'Annual age-grouping and athlete development: a meta-analytical review of relative age effects in sport', *Sports Medicine*, 39(3): 235–56.

Cohen, J. (1960) 'A coefficient of agreement for nominal scales', *Educational and Psychological Measurement*, 20: 37–46.

Cohen, L., Manion, L. and Morrison, K. (2011) *Research Methods in Education*, 7th edn, London: Routledge.

Coleclough, J. (2013), 'Soccer coaches' and referees' perceptions of tackle incidents with respect to the laws of the game', *International Journal of Performance Analysis in Sport*, 13: 553–66.

Cooter, M. (2009) Style: what is it and why does it matter. In G.M. Hall (ed.), *How to Write a Scientific Paper*, 4th edn (pp. 117–22), Oxford: Wiley-Blackwell.

Cort, M. (2006) 'Voice activated data entry and performance analysis: going back to the future'. In H. Dancs, M. Hughes and P.G. O'Donoghue (eds), *Performance Analysis of Sport 7* (pp. 87–8), Cardiff, UK: UWIC CPA Press.

Coutts, A.J. and Duffield, R. (2010) 'Validity and reliability of GPS devices for measuring movement demands of team sports', *Journal of Science and Medicine in Sport*, 13: 133–5.

Creme, P. and Lea, M.R. (2008) *Writing at University: A guide for Students*, 3rd edn, Maidenhead, UK: Open University Press/McGraw-Hill.

Csataljay, G., O'Donoghue, P.G., Hughes, M.D. and Dancs, H. (2009) 'Performance indicators that distinguish winning and losing teams in basketball', *International Journal of Performance Analysis of Sport*, 9: 60–6.

Curran, P., O'Donoghue, P.G., Jackson, K., Hull, M.E.C. and Griffiths, L. (1994) 'BORIS-R specification of the requirements of a large scale software intensive system', Workshop on Requirements Elicitation for Software-based Systems, Keele, 12–14 July.

Di Felice, U. and Marcora, S. (2013) 'Errors in judging Olympic boxing performance: false negative or false positive'. In D. Peters and P.G. O'Donoghue (eds), *Performance Analysis of Sport IX* (pp. 190–5), London: Routledge.

Di Salvo, V., Gregson, W., Atkinson, G., Tordoff, P. and Drust, B. (2009) 'Analysis of high intensity activity in Premier League soccer', *International Journal of Sports Medicine*, 30: 205–12.

Donnelly, C. and O'Donoghue, P.G. (2008) 'Behaviour of netball coaches of different levels', paper presented at the World Congress of Performance Analysis of Sport 8, Magdeburg, 3–6 September 2008.

D'Ottavio, S. and Castagna, C. (2001) 'Physiological load imposed on elite soccer referees during actual match play', *Journal of Sports Medicine and Physical Fitness*, 41: 27–32.

Dowrick, P.W. (1991) *Practical Guide to Using Video in the Behavioural Sciences*, New York: John Wiley and Sons.

Dowrick, P.W. and Raeburn, J.M. (1977) 'Video editing and medication to produce a therapeutic self-model', *Journal of Consulting in Clinical Psychology*, 45: 1156–8.

Dufour, W. (1991) 'Computer assisted scouting in soccer'. In J. Clarys, T. Reilly and A. Stibbe (eds), *Science and Football II* (pp.160–6), London: E. and F.N. Spon.

Evans, J. (1986) *The Complete Guide to Windsurfing*, London: Bell and Hyman.

Franks, I.M. (1997) 'Use of feedback by coaches and players'. In T. Reilly, J. Bangsbo and M. Hughes (eds), *Science and Football 3* (pp. 267–78), London: E. and F.N. Spon.

Franks, I.M. and Goodman, D. (1984) 'A hierarchical approach to performance analysis', *SPORTS*, June.

Franks, I.M. and Miller, G. (1986) 'Eyewitness testimony in sport', *Journal of Sport Behaviour*, 9: 39–45.

Franks, I.M. and Miller, G. (1991) 'Training coaches to observe and remember', *Journal of Sports Sciences*, 9: 285–97.

Franks, I.M., Goodman, D. and Miller, G. (1983) 'Human factors in sports systems: an empirical investigation of events in team games', Proceedings of the Human Factors Society – twenty-seventh annual meeting, pp. 383–6.

Gangstead, S.K. and Beveridge S.K. (1984) 'The implementation and evaluation of a methodological approach to qualitative sportskill analysis instruction', *Journal of Teaching Physical Education*, Winter: 60–70.

Gerisch, G. and Reichelt, M. (1993) 'Computer and video aided analysis of football games'. In T. Reilly, J. Clarys and A. Stibbe (eds), *Science and Football II* (pp. 167–74). London: E. & F.N. Spon.

Gomez, M.A., Lagos-Peñas, C. and Pollard, R. (2013) 'Situational variables'. In T. McGarry, P.G. O'Donoghue and J. Sampaio (eds), *Routledge Handbook of Sports Performance Analysis* (pp. 259–69), London: Routledge.

Greene, D., Leyshon, W. and O'Donoghue, P.G. (2008) 'Elite male 400m hurdle tactics are influenced by race leader', paper presented at the World Congress of Performance Analysis of Sport 8, Magdeburg, 3–6 September 2008.

Greenlees, I., Leyland, A., Thelwell, R. and Filey, W. (2008) 'Soccer penalty takers' uniform colour and pre-penalty kick gaze affect the impressions formed of them by opposing goalkeepers', *Journal of Sports Sciences*, 26: 569–76.

Gregson, W., Drust, B., Atkinson, G. and Salvo, V.D. (2010) 'Match-to-match variability of high-speed activities in Premier League soccer', *International Journal of Sports Medicine*, 31: 237–42.

Grehaigne, J.F., Bouthier, D. and David, B. (1997) 'A method to analyse attacking moves in soccer'. In T. Reilly, J. Bangsbo and M. Hughes (eds), *Science and Football III* (pp. 258–64), London: E. & F.N. Spon.

Gustavii, B. (2008) *How to Write and Illustrate a Scientific Paper*, 2nd edn, Cambridge: Cambridge University Press.

Hale, S. (2004) 'Work-rate of Welsh national league players in training matches and competitive matches'. In P.G. O'Donoghue and M. Hughes (eds), *Performance Analysis of Sport 6* (pp. 35–44), Cardiff: CPA Press, UWIC.

Hall, G.M. (2009) 'Structure of a scientific paper'. In G.M. Hall (ed.), *How to Write a Scientific Paper*, 4th edn (pp. 1–4), Oxford: Wiley-Blackwell.

Harries, N. and O'Donoghue, P.G. (2012) 'A temporal analysis of combinations in professional boxing', *International Journal of Performance Analysis in Sport*, 12: 707.

Hay, J.G. and Reid, J.G. (1988) *Anatomy, Mechanics and Human Motion*, Englewood Cliffs, NJ: Prentice-Hall.

Hayes, M. (1997) 'When is research not research? When it's notational analysis', *BASES Newsletter*, 7(7): 4–5.

Hibbs, A. and O'Donoghue, P.G. (2013) 'Strategy and tactics in sports performance'. In T. McGarry, P.G. O'Donoghue and J. Sampaio (eds), *Routledge Handbook of Sports Performance Analysis* (248–58), London: Routledge.

Horwill, F. (1991) *Obsession for Running: A Lifetime in Athletics*, Carnforth, UK: Colin Davis Printers.

Huey, A., Morrow, P. and O'Donoghue, P.G. (2001) 'From time-motion analysis to specific intermittent high intensity training'. In M. Hughes and I.M. Franks (eds), *Performance Analysis, Sports Science and Computers* (pp. 29–34), Cardiff: CPA Press, UWIC.

Hughes, M. (1998) 'The application of notational analysis to racket sports'. In A. Lees, I. Maynard, M. Hughes and T. Reilly (eds), *Science and Racket Sports 2* (pp. 211–20), London: E. and F.N. Spon.

Hughes, M.D. (2008) 'Notational analysis for coaches'. In R.L. Jones, M. Hughes and K. Kingston (eds), *An Introduction to Sports Coaching: From Science and Theory to Practice* (pp. 101–13), London: Routledge.

248

Hughes, M. and Bartlett, R. (2002) 'The use of performance indicators in performance analysis', *Journal of Sports Sciences*, 20: 739–54.

Hughes, M. and Bartlett, R. (2004) 'The use of performance indicators in performance analysis'. In M.D. Hughes and I.M. Franks (eds), *Notational Analysis of Sport,: Systems for Better Coaching and Performance in Sport*, 2nd edn (pp. 166–88), London: Routledge.

Hughes, M. and Bartlett, R. (2008) 'What is performance analysis?' In M. Hughes and I.M. Franks (eds), *Essentials of Performance Analysis: An Introduction* (pp. 8–20), London: Routledge.

Hughes, M. and Clarke, S. (1995) 'Surface effect on elite tennis strategy', In T. Reilly, M. Hughes and A. Lees (eds), *Science and Racket Sports* (pp. 272–7), London: E. and F.N. Spon.

Hughes, M. and Franks, I.M. (1995) 'History of notational analysis of soccer', Keynote address, Third World Congress of Science and Football, Cardiff, 9–13 April 1995.

Hughes, M. and Franks, I.M. (2004a) 'Literature review'. In M. Hughes and I.M. Franks (eds), *Notational Analysis of Sport,: Systems for Better Coaching and Performance in Sport*, 2nd edn, (pp. 59–106), London: Routledge.

Hughes, M. and Franks, I.M. (2004b) 'Sports analysis'. In M. Hughes and I.M. Franks (eds), *Notational Analysis of Sport,: Systems for Better Coaching and Performance in Sport*, 2nd edn, (pp. 107–17), London: Routledge.

Hughes, M. and Franks, I.M. (2004c) 'How to develop a notation system'. In M. Hughes and I.M. Franks (eds), *Notational Analysis of Sport,: Systems for Better Coaching and Performance in Sport*, 2nd edn,(pp. 118–40), London: Routledge.

Hughes, M. and Franks, I.M. (2004d) 'Examples of notation systems'. In M. Hughes and I.M. Franks (eds), *Notational Analysis of Sport,: Systems for Better Coaching and Performance in Sport*, 2nd edn, (pp. 141–87), London: Routledge.

Hughes, M. and Franks, I.M. (2005) 'Analysis of passing sequences, shots and goals in soccer', *Journal of Sports Sciences*, 23: 509–14.

Hughes, M., Cooper, S.M. and Nevill, A. (2004) 'Analysis of notation data: reliability'. In M. Hughes and I.M. Franks (eds), *Notational Analysis of Sport,: Systems for Better Coaching and Performance in Sport*, 2nd edn, (pp. 189–204), London: Routledge.

Hughes, M.G., Rose, G. and Amaral, I. (2005) 'The influence of recovery duration on blood lactate accumulation in repeated sprint activity', *Journal of Sports Sciences*, 23: 130–1.

Hunter, P. and O'Donoghue, P.G. (2001) 'A match analysis of the 1999 Rugby Union World Cupp. In M. Hughes and I.M. Franks (eds), *Proceedings of the World Congress of Performance Analysis, Sports Science and Computers (PASS.COM)* (pp. 85–90), Cardiff: CPA Press, UWIC.

James, N., Jones, N.M.P. and Hollely, C. (2002) 'Reliability of selected performance analysis systems in football and rugby', Proceedings of the Fourth International Conference on Methods and Techniques in Behavioural Research. Amsterdam: The Netherlands, pp. 116–8.

James, N. (2008) 'Performance analysis in the media'. In M. Hughes and I.M.

Franks (eds), *The Essentials of Performance Analysis: An Introduction* (pp. 243–63), London: Routledge.

Johnson, C. (1984) *Hammer Throwing*, London: British Amateur Athletic Board.

Johns, P. and Brouner, J. (2013) 'The efficacy of judging within trampolining'. In D. Peters and P.G. O'Donoghue (eds), *Performance Analysis of Sport IX* (pp. 214–21), London: Routledge.

Kirkbride, A. (2013a) 'Scoring/judging applications'. In T. McGarry, P.G. O'Donoghue and J. Sampaio (eds), *Routledge Handbook of Sports Performance Analysis* (pp. 140–52), London: Routledge.

Kirkbride, A. (2013b) 'Media applications of performance analysis'. In T. McGarry, P.G. O'Donoghue and J. Sampaio (eds), *Routledge Handbook of Sports Performance Analysis* (pp. 187–90), London: Routledge.

Knight, G. and O'Donoghue, P.G. (2012) 'The probability of winning break points in Grand Slam men's singles tennis', *European Journal of Sports Science*, 12: 462–8.

Knudson, D.V. (2013) *Qualitative Diagnosis of Human movement*, 3rd edn, Champaign, IL: Human Kinetics.

Knudson, D.V. and Morrison, C.S. (2002) *Qualitative Analysis of Human Movement*, 2nd edn, Champaign, IL: Human Kinetics.

Koon Teck, K., Wang, C.K.J. and Mallett, C.J. (2012) 'Discriminating factors between successful and unsuccessful elite youth Olympic female basketball teams', *International Journal of Performance Analysis in Sport*, 12: 119–31.

Lacy, A.C. and Darst, P.W. (1984) 'Evolution of a systematic observation system: the ASU coaching observation instrument', *Journal of Teaching in Physical Education*, 3: 59–66.

Lacy, A.C. and Darst, P.W. (1985) 'Systematic observation of behaviour of winning high school head football coaches', *Journal of Teaching in Physical Education*, 4: 256–70.

Lacy, A.C. and Darst, P.W. (1989) 'The Arizona State University Observation Instrument (ASUOI)'. In P.W. Darst, D.B. Zakrajsek and V.H. Mancini (eds), *Analysing Physical Education and Sport Instruction,* 2nd edn (pp. 369–77), Champaign, IL: Human Kinetics.

Lafont, D. (2007) 'Towards a new hitting model in tennis', *International Journal of Performance Analysis of Sport*, 7(3): 106–16.

Lafont, D. (2008) 'Gaze control during the hitting phase in tennis: a preliminary study', *International Journal of Performance Analysis of Sport*, 8(1): 85–100.

Laird, P. and Waters, L. (2008) 'Eye-witness recollection of sports coaches', *International Journal of Performance Analysis of Sport*, 8(1): 76–84.

Larkin, P., Berry, J., Dawson, B. and Lay, B. (2011) 'Perceptual and decision-making skills of Australian football umpires', *International Journal of Performance Analysis in Sport*, 11: 427–37.

Lees, A. (2008) 'Qualitative biomechanical analysis of technique'. In M. Hughes and I.M. Franks (eds), *The Essentials of Performance Analysis: An Introduction* (pp. 162–79). London: Routledge.

Leser, R. and Kwon, Y.-H. (2014 in press) 'Computer video systems', in A.Baca (ed.), *Sports Informatics*, London: Routledge.

Leyshon, W. (2012) 'Performance analysis in the management of high performance sport – international 400m hurdles', Keynote presentation, World Congress of Performance Analysis of Sport IX, Worcester, UK, 25–28 July 2012.

Liddle, S.D., Murphy, M.H. and Bleakley, E.W. (1996) 'A comparison of the demands of singles and doubles badminton among elite male players: a heart rate and time-motion analysis', *Journal of Human Movement Studies*, 29(4): 159–76.

Lorenzo, A., Gomez, M.A., Ortega, E., Ibañez, S. J. and Sampaio, J. (2010) 'Game related statistics which discriminate between winning and losing under-16 male basketball games', *Journal of Sports Science and Medicine*, 9(4): 664–8.

Lupo, C., Capranica, L., Ammendolia, A., Rizzuto, F. and Tessitore, A. (2012) 'Performance analysis in youth waterbasket – a physiological, time motion, and notational analysis of a new aquatic team sport', *International Journal of Performance Analysis in Sport*, 12: 1–13.

Marinho, D.A., Barbosa, T.M., Neiva, H.P., Costa, M.J., Garrido, M.D. and Silva, A.J. (2013) 'Swimming, running, cycling and triathlon'. In T. McGarry, P.G. O'Donoghue and J. Sampaio (eds), *Routledge Handbook of Sports Performance Analysis* (pp. 436–63), London: Routledge.

Matthews, J.R. and Matthews, R.W. (2008) *Successful Scientific Writing: A Step-by-step Guide for the Biological and Medical Sciences*, 3rd edn, Cambridge: Cambridge University Press.

Mayes, A., O'Donoghue, P.G., Garland, J. and Davidson, A. (2009) 'The use of performance analysis and internet video streaming during elite netball preparation', *International Journal of Performance Analysis of Sport*, 9(3): 435.

McCorry, M., Saunders, E.D., O'Donoghue, P.G. and Murphy, M.H. (1996) 'A match analysis of the knockout stages of the 3rd Rugby Union World Cup'. In M. Hughes (ed.), *Notational Analysis of Sport 3* (pp. 230–9), Cardiff: CPA Press, UWIC.

McGarry, T., O'Donoghue, P.G. and Sampaio, J. (2013), *Routledge Handbook of Sports Performance Analysis* (pp. 436–63), London: Routledge.

MacKenzie, R. and Cushion, C. (2013) 'Performance analysis in football: a critical review and implications for future research', *Journal of Sports Sciences*, 31: 639–76.

McLaughlin, E. and O'Donoghue, P.G. (2001) 'The reliability of time-motion analysis using the CAPTAIN system'. In M. Hughes and I.M. Franks (eds), *Proceedings of the World Congress of Performance Analysis, Sports Science and Computers (PASS.COM)* (pp. 63–8), Cardiff: CPA Press, UWIC.

McNair, D.M., Lorr, M. and Droppelman, L. (1971) *Manual: Profile of Mood States*, San Diego, CA: Educational and Industrial Testing Service Inc.

Mellick, M. (2005) 'Elite referee decision communication: developing a model of best practice'. Unpublished PhD Thesis, University of Wales Institute Cardiff.

Mizohata, J., O'Donoghue, P.G. and Hughes, M. (2009) 'Work-rate of senior rugby union referees during matches', *International Journal of Performance Analysis in Sport*, 9(3): 436.

Mullan, A. and O'Donoghue, P.G. (2001) 'An alternative computerised scoring system for amateur boxing'. In M. Hughes and I.M. Franks (eds), *Proceedings of the World Congress of Performance Analysis, Sports Science and Computers (PASS.COM)* (pp. 359–64), Cardiff: CPA Press, UWIC.

Norman, D.A. and Draper S.W. (1986), *User Centred System Design*, Hillsdale, NJ: Lawrence Erlbaum.

Nunome, H., Drust, B. and Dawson, B. (2013), *Science and Football VII*, London: Routledge.

O'Donoghue, PG. (1998) 'Time-motion analysis of work-rate in elite soccer'. In M. Hughes and F. Tavares (eds), *Notational Analysis of Sport 4* (pp. 65–70). Porto: University of Porto.

O'Donoghue, P.G. (2002) 'Performance models of ladies' and men's singles tennis at the Australian Open', *International Journal of Performance Analysis of Sport*, 2: 73–84.

O'Donoghue, P.G. (2005a) 'Normative profiles of sports performance', *International Journal of Performance Analysis of Sport*, 5(1): 104–19.

O'Donoghue, P.G. (2005b) 'An algorithm to use the kappa statistic to establish reliability of computerised time-motion analysis systems', *Book of Abstracts, FifthInternational Symposium of Computer Science in Sport*, Hvar, Croatia, 25–28 May, p.49.

O'Donoghue, P.G. (2008a) 'Time-motion analysis'. In M. Hughes and I.M. Franks (eds), *Essentials of Performance Analysis: An Introduction* (pp. 180–205). London: Routledge.

O'Donoghue, P.G. (2009) 'Interacting performances theory', *International Journal of Performance Analysis of Sport*, 9: 26–46.

O'Donoghue, P.G. (2010) *Research Methods for Sports Performance Analysis*, London: Routledge.

O'Donoghue, P.G. (2012) 'Strategy in national championship 2000m indoor rowing', *International Journal of Performance Analysis in* Sport, 12: 809.

O'Donoghue, P.G. (2013a) 'Match analysis for coaches'. In R.L. Jones and K. Kingston (eds), *An Introduction to Sports Coaching: Connecting Theory to Practice*, 2nd edn (pp. 161–75), London: Routledge.

O'Donoghue, P.G. (2013b) 'Rare events in tennis', *International Journal of Performance Analysis in Sport*, 13: 535–52.

O'Donoghue, P.G. and Holmes, L. (2015) *Data Analysis in Sport*, London: Routledge.

O'Donoghue, P.G. and Ingram, B. (2001) 'A notational analysis of elite tennis strategy', *Journal of Sports Sciences*, 19: 107–15.

O'Donoghue, P.G. and Liddle, S.D. (1998) 'A notational analysis of time factors of elite men's and ladies' singles tennis on clay and grass surfaces'. In A. Lees, I. Maynard, M. Hughes and T. Reilly (eds), *Science and Racket Sports 2* (pp. 241–6), London: E. & F.N. Spon.

O'Donoghue, P.G. and Longville, J. (2004) 'Reliability testing and the use of statistics in performance analysis support: a case study from an international netball tournament'. In P.G. O'Donoghue and M. Hughes (eds), *Performance Analysis of Sport 6* (pp. 1–7), Cardiff: CPA Press, UWIC.

O'Donoghue, P.G. and Mayes, A. (2013a) 'Performance analysis, feedback and communication in coaching'. In T. McGarry, P.G. O'Donoghue and J. Sampaio (eds), *Routledge Handbook of Sports Performance Analysis* (pp. 155–64), London: Routledge.

O'Donoghue, P.G. and Mayes, A. (2013b) 'Coach behaviour'. In T. McGarry, P.G.

O'Donoghue and J. Sampaio (eds), *Routledge Handbook of Sports Performance Analysis* (pp. 165–74), London: Routledge.

O'Donoghue, P.G. and Parker, D. (2001) 'Time-motion analysis of FA Premier League soccer competition'. In M. Hughes and I.M. Franks (eds), *Proceedings of the World Congress of Performance Analysis, Sports Science and Computers (PASS.COM)* (pp. 263–6), Cardiff: CPA Press, UWIC.

O'Donoghue, P.G. and Robinson, G. (2009) 'Validation of the ProZone3® player tracking system: a preliminary report', *International Journal of Computer Science in Sport*, 8(1): 38–53.

O'Donoghue, P.G., Hughes, M.G., Rudkin, S., Bloomfield, J., Cairns, G. and Powell, S. (2005a) 'Work-rate analysis using the POWER (Periods of Work Efforts and Recoveries) System', *International Journal of Performance Analysis of Sport*, 4(1): 5–21.

O'Donoghue, P.G., Rudkin, S., Bloomfield, J., Powell, S., Cairns, G., Dunkerley, A., Davey, P., Probert, G. and Bowater, J. (2005b) 'Repeated work activity in English FA Premier League soccer', *International Journal of Performance Analysis of Sport*, 5(2): 46–57.

Olsen, E. and Larsen, O. (1997) 'Use of match analysis by coaches'. In T. Reilly, J. Bangsbo and M. Hughes (eds), *Science and Football 3* (pp. 209–20), London: E. & F.N. Spon.

Palao, J.M. and Morante, J.C. (2013) 'Technical effectiveness'. In T. McGarry, P.G. O'Donoghue and J. Sampaio (eds), *Routledge Handbook of Sports Performance Analysis* (pp. 213–24), London: Routledge.

Pedemonte, J. (1985) 'Hammer'. In H. Payne (ed), *Athletes in Action: The Official International Amateur Athletic Federation Book on Track and Field Techniques* (pp. 237–62), London: Pelham Books.

Peters, D.M. and O'Donoghue, P.G. (2013) *Performance Analysis of Sport IX*, London: Routledge.

Petersen, C. and Dawson, B. (2013) 'Cricket'. In T. McGarry, P.G. O'Donoghue and J. Sampaio (eds), *Routledge Handbook of Sports Performance Analysis* (pp. 393–403), London: Routledge.

Poziat, G., Adé, D., Seifert, L., Trousaint, H. and Gal-Petitfaux, N. (2010) 'Evaluation of the measuring active drag system usability: an important step for its integration into training sessions', *International Journal of Performance Analysis in Sport*, 10: 170–86.

Poziat, G., Sève, C. and Saury, J. (2013) 'Qualitative aspects in performance'. In T. McGarry, P.G. O'Donoghue and J. Sampaio (eds), *Routledge Handbook of Sports Performance Analysis* (pp. 309–20), London: Routledge.

Priebe, H-J. (2009) 'Results'. In G.M. Hall (ed.), *How to Write a Scientific Paper*, 4th edn (pp. 19–30),Oxford: Wiley-Blackwell.

Pyle, I., Hruschka, P., Lissandra, M. and Jackson, K. (1993) *Real-time Systems: Investigating Industrial Practice*, Chichester, UK: John Wiley & Sons Ltd.

Rampinini, E., Impellizzeri, F.M., Castagna, C., Coutts, A.J. and Wisløff, U. (2009) 'Technical performance during soccer matches of the Italian Serie A league: effect of fatigue and competitive level', *Journal of Science and Medicine in Sport*, 12(1): 227–33.

Redwood-Brown, A., O'Donoghue, P.G. and Robinson, G. 'The interaction effect of positional role and scoreline on work-rate in FA Premier League soccer', paper presented at the Third International Workshop of the International Society of Performance Analysis of Sport, Lincoln, 6–7 April 2009.

Redwood-Brown, A., O'Donoghue, P.G., Robinson, G. and Neilson, P. (2012) 'The effect of score-line on work-rate in English FA Premier League soccer', *International Journal of Performance Analysis in Sport*, 12: 258–71.

Reid, M., McMurtrie, D. and Crespo, M. (2010) 'The relationship between match statistics and top 100 ranking in professional men's tennis', *International Journal of Performance Analysis in Sport*, 10: 131–8.

Reilly, T. and Thomas, V. (1976) 'A motion analysis of work rate in different positional roles in professional football match play', *Journal of Human Movement Studies*, 2: 87–97.

Robinson, P. (1992) *HOOD: Hierarchical Object Oriented Design*, Englewood Cliffs, NJ: Prentice-Hall.

Robinson, G., O'Donoghue, P.G. and Nielson, P. (2011), 'Path changes and injury risk in English FA Premier League soccer', *International Journal of Performance Analysis in Sport*, 11: 40–56.

Rose-Doherty, E. and O'Donoghue, P.G. (2012) 'Accuracy of netball umpiring in the British National Super League', *International Journal of Performance Analysis in Sport*, 12: 697.

Schön, D.A. (1983) *The Reflective Practitioner. How Professionals Think in Action*, London: Temple Smith.

Siegle, M. and Lames, M. (2010), 'The relation between movement velocity and movement pattern in elite soccer', *International Journal of Performance Analysis in Sport*, 10: 270–8.

Smith, R. (2009) 'Introduction'. In G.M. Hall (ed.), *How to Write a Scientific Paper*, 4th edn (pp. 5–13), Oxford: Wiley-Blackwell.

Sommerville, I. (1992) *Software Engineering*, 4th edn, Wokingham, UK: Addison-Wesley.

Spencer, M., Lawrence, S., Rechichi, C., Bishop, D., Dawson, B. and Goodman, C. (2004) 'Time-motion analysis of elite field hockey, with special reference to repeated-sprint activity', *Journal of Sports Sciences*, 22: 843–50.

Taylor, S. and Hughes, M. (1988) 'Computerised notational analysis: a voice interactive system', *Journal of Sports Sciences*, 6: 255.

Taylor, J.B., Mellalieu, S.D., James, N. and Shearer, U.A. (2008) 'The influence of match location, quality of opposition and match status on technical performance in professional association football', *Journal of Sports Sciences*, 26: 885–95.

Theureau, J. (2003) 'Course of action analysis and course of action centred design'. In E. Hollnagel (ed.), *Handbook of Cognitive Task Design* (pp. 55–81), Mahwah, NJ: Lawrence Erlbaum.

Vaz, L., Mouchet, A., Carreras, D. and Morente, H. (2011) 'The importance of rugby game-related statistics to discriminate winners and losers at the elite level competitions in close and balanced games', *International Journal of Performance Analysis in Sport*, 11: 130–41.

Walliman, N. (2004) *Your Undergraduate Dissertation: The Essential Guide*, London: Sage.

254

Williams, J.J. (2004) 'The development of a real-time data capture application for rugby union'. In P.G. O'Donoghue and M.D. Hughes (eds), *Performance Analysis of Sport VI* (pp. 253–61), Cardiff: UWIC CPA Press.

Williams, R. and O'Donoghue, P. (2005) 'Lower limb injury risk in netball: a time-motion analysis investigation', *Journal of Human Movement Studies*, 49: 315–31.

Williams, N. and O'Donoghue, P.G. (2006) 'Techniques used in mixed-martial arts competition', *Performance Analysis of Sport 7* (edited by H. Dancs, M. Hughes and P.G. O'Donoghue), 23–26 August, Szombathely, Hungary, Cardiff: CPA UWIC Press, pp. 393–9.

Wiltshire, H.D. (2013) 'Sports performance analysis for high performance managers'. In T. McGarry, P.G. O'Donoghue and J. Sampaio (eds), *Routledge Handbook of Sports Performance Analysis* (pp. 176–86), London: Routledge.

Winkler, W. (1988) 'A new approach to the video analysis of tactical aspects of soccer'. In T. Reilly, A. Lees, K. Davids and W. Murphy (eds), *Science and Football* (pp. 368–72), London: E. & F.N. Spon.

Withers, R.T., Maricic, Z., Wasilewski, S. and Kelly, L. (1982) 'Match analysis of Australian professional soccer players', *Journal of Human Movement Studies*, 8: 158–76.

Wright, B., Rodenberg, R.M. and Sackmann, J. (2013) 'Incentives in best of N Contests: quasi-Simpson's paradox in tennis', *International Journal of Performance Analysis in Sport*, 13: 790–802.

# INDEX

256

258

**259**

260